PRAIS

"*Get It Out* is an essential read for all who care for bodies with and without uteruses, and those who want to liberate reproductive freedoms and protect bodily autonomy in medicine."
—Renee Bracey Sherman, coauthor of *Liberating Abortion: Claiming Our History, Sharing Our Stories, and Building the Reproductive Future We Deserve*

"*Get It Out* offers an urgent intervention in lasting reproductive health inequalities. Examining the complicated narratives of cisgender women, trans, and nonbinary people who have had—or are considering having—a hysterectomy, Becker astutely shows how health access and experiences are shaped along the social fault lines of race, class, and gender."
—stef m. shuster, author of *Trans Medicine: The Emergence and Practice of Treating Gender*

"A highly accessible and nuanced account of hysterectomy that traces its social underpinnings and reveals the continued operation of reproductive stratification along race and gender lines."
—Krystale E. Littlejohn, author of *Just Get on the Pill: The Uneven Burden of Reproductive Politics*

"A new, surprising, and essential read in the wake of Dobbs, *Get It Out* will change how you think about the uterus."
—Moira Donegan, journalist and host of *In Bed with the Right*

"Becker probes the complicated, sometimes violent, and sometimes life-saving history of hysterectomy. The interviews in this book are deeply human—full of pain, fury, and relief. Altogether, they suggest a vision of the future in which everyone has the freedom to choose hysterectomy, and, by extension, the right of self-determination."
—Sabrina Imbler, author of *How Far the Light Reaches: A Life in Ten Sea Creatures*

GET IT OUT

HEALTH, SOCIETY, AND INEQUALITY SERIES

General Editor: Jennifer A. Reich

GET IT OUT

ON THE POLITICS OF HYSTERECTOMY

ANDRÉA BECKER

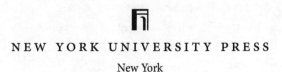

NEW YORK UNIVERSITY PRESS

New York

NEW YORK UNIVERSITY PRESS
New York
www.nyupress.org

Please contact the Library of Congress for Cataloging-in-Publication data.
ISBN: 9781479826599 (hardback)
ISBN: 9781479826605 (paperback)
ISBN: 9781479826643 (library ebook)
ISBN: 9781479826629 (consumer ebook)

This book is printed on acid-free paper, and its binding materials are chosen for strength and durability. We strive to use environmentally responsible suppliers and materials to the greatest extent possible in publishing our books.

The manufacturer's authorized representative in the EU for product safety is Mare Nostrum Group B.V., Mauritskade 21D, 1091 GC Amsterdam, The Netherlands. Email: gpsr@mare-nostrum.co.uk.

Manufactured in the United States of America

10 9 8 7 6 5 4 3 2 1

Also available as an ebook

CONTENTS

AUTHOR'S NOTE

> There are parts of your own body less known than
> the bottom of the ocean or the surface of Mars.
> —Rachel E. Gross, *Vagina Obscura:*
> *An Anatomical Voyage*

This book is dedicated to the uterus—a misunderstood organ, an organ dubbed "the origin of all disease" in Hippocratic texts, the organ we all once called home. Though only the size of a fist, it's been forced to hold impossibly large societal questions and controversies. The uterus is a cultural battleground on which to debate where life begins, a woman's right to choose, how much pain is ordinary pain, and what it means to align your body to match your gender. I dedicate this book to every scientist, every writer, every doctor, every policymaker, every person working to shed light on the needlessly mysterious ways of the uterus and to improve life for the people who have them.

Many with uteruses were taught to feel shame about this organ and its manifold functions. I, for one, was taught to hide my tampon wrappers in tissue, lest my male relatives be forced to see the evidence of my menstruation in the trash can of our shared bathroom—evidence that I have a uterus, an organ that bleeds. Many grew up saying phrases like "lady parts," "down there," and "my time of the month," and even those of us who menstruate every month weren't taught to fully understand the menstrual cycle, including the differences between menstruation and ovulation and the names of the hormones involved in these twin processes. The medical and scientific communities reflect this censoring and lack of knowing amid countless gaps in research and treatments. There are five times more studies on erectile dysfunction than there are on premenstrual syndrome (PMS), for instance, even though over 90 percent of people with uteruses experience PMS.[1] We have known about uterus-adjacent diseases like endometriosis and fibroids for more than a hundred years, yet without adequate research, these highly common illnesses remain mysterious and difficult to treat. It is within this lack of knowing about the uterus that shame seeps in.

This book is dedicated to everyone who struggles with their uterus—or lack thereof. To everyone whose uterine pain has been minimized by doctors, parents, peers, and teachers. To everyone who had ailments of pain that went undiagnosed for years. To everyone who wishes they never had a uterus to begin with. To everyone who wishes they *were* born with a uterus. To everyone who longs for a uterus that can carry a healthy pregnancy to term. There are countless unanswered questions about the uterus, but with every story told, we are a step closer to understanding this unnecessarily black box.

It has been an honor to be tasked with collecting and recording the uterus stories in this book—stories that, like the uterus itself, reflect strength, resilience, and regeneration.

INTRODUCTION

"NOT YOUR MOTHER'S HYSTERECTOMY"

That fist-shaped muscle, that powerful source, that place
where we all began. It might even tell us, in so many ways,
where we are all going.
— Leah Hazard, *Womb: The Inside Story
of Where We All Began*

Having a uterus is a relentless job. Even those with a purportedly easy, regular menstrual period find themselves inundated with administrative tasks once a month: anticipate the bleeding, reduce the pain, buy more tampons, wash the menstrual cup, scrub red out of fabric. Then there are the 10 percent of people with a uterus who have endometriosis, a disease that researchers have known about since the early twentieth century and yet is still widely considered a medical enigma with no cure. Even today, patients wait about a decade on average to receive a formal diagnosis—which can only happen through surgery.[1] Add adenomyosis, fibroids, uterine prolapse, gender dysphoria, and polycystic ovary syndrome (PCOS) to the list, and the share of people with uteruses for whom at least a week out of every month is hell grows. And then there's avoiding pregnancy: demanding, thankless work that occupies thirty consecutive years on average, ranging from a tedious daily pill to the dreadful placing of an intrauterine device (IUD).[2] All the while, any pain, discomfort, or side effects involved in these bodily experiences and projects are normalized, minimized, denied, or ignored—deemed part and parcel of occupying a body of this sort. If housework and childcare constitute the "second shift" after the workday for women,[3] then simply having a uterus is the shift that never ends.

It is no wonder, then, that having one's uterus removed via hysterectomy is an attractive prospect to some. It is so attractive, in fact, that six hundred thousand hysterectomies are performed each year—at least one hysterectomy for every minute of the year—making it the most frequently performed gynecological surgery worldwide.[4] Within the United States alone, a fifth of those born with a uterus will have it removed by the age of sixty-five.[5]

Hysterectomies can be traced back as early as 50 BC, but the modern hysterectomy is now largely regarded as a minimally invasive, typically outpatient procedure that leaves behind tiny abdominal scars.[6] Given the vast advancements in hysterectomy techniques, this surgery now fits into the cultural zeitgeist of using medical tools to enhance one's quality of life. We live in an age of "biohacking" or "technofixing," where individuals work to optimize the performance, appearance, and longevity of the human body. Within the broad landscape of nutritional supplements, reconstructive and cosmetic surgeries, lifestyle modifications, and the second-to-second tracking of our own bodily data with Fitbits and Apple watches, it seems only natural that a person whose uterus is underperforming would want a hysterectomy. In this light, a hysterectomy can techno-fix or optimize one's body by excising pain, bleeding, and even the need for birth control. As increasing numbers of Americans desire to be child-free or have begun to decouple gender and family from body parts, the procedure's benefits appear to outweigh any purported losses. Nonetheless, the core assumption that hysterectomy is a necessary evil that thrusts infertility onto people overshadows these alternative understandings.

Although hysterectomy is extremely common, the procedure has been highly understudied, particularly within the social sciences. What we *do* know about hysterectomy tends to link the surgery with oppressive medical overreach that increases rather than alleviates suffering. Historians, theorists, activists, and medical practitioners largely discuss hysterectomy as an unnecessary procedure forced upon women by "hyster-happy" practitioners.[7] This has occurred both contemporarily,[8] as well as throughout history.[9] Admittedly, hysterectomy tends to problematically be the catchall solution offered for all uterus-inflicted maladies, since few alternatives exist that provide permanent cures for diseases of the uterus. Yet, cultural conceptions of hysterectomy are funneled through this lens of anti-woman, physician-inflicted suffering, even when it is a legitimate solution that can improve lives. A quick Google search for "hysterectomy book," for instance, provides hair-raising results like *The Hysterectomy Hoax*, *Do You Really Need Surgery?*, and *The Castrated Woman*, and *No*

More Hysterectomies.[10] Looking within the field of sociology, my own field and where the idea for this book began, the sole book wholly dedicated to hysterectomy is titled *Am I Still a Woman?*[11]

With this book, and as a medical sociologist interested in the "contested" realms of healthcare, I aim to figure out what it means to *choose* a modern, technologically refined hysterectomy in today's world—one that simultaneously encourages technofixing of bodies but shuns hysterectomies. Hysterectomy is exemplary of the ways in which all reproductive health choices are constrained within inter-locking systems of inequality. After all, hysterectomy involves a key reproductive organ associated with or, often, used as *the* symbol for, women, and any such procedure tends to become a symbolic reposi-tory for cultural anxieties about gender, the family, race, and even the health of society. Hysterectomy is a heightened, permanent way to not only make the choice not to be pregnant (*against* childbearing) but also not to be able to be pregnant (to opt *into* infertility in the service of other goals). Central to this book's focus, therefore, is the question of what choosing really means and entails, if hysterectomy is at all choosable.

Moral panics emerge and proliferate around any healthcare that disrupts "female reproduction," including less permanent forms of reproductive disruption like contraceptives and abortion—both of which are already subject to increasingly polarizing discourses and legislative attacks. Hysterectomy, by rendering future gestation im-possible, produces particular cultural anxieties. It calls into question the mutability of bodies and the increasing role of medicine and tech-nology: If people can readily remove the very organ that society has used to denote their otherness, how will the gender order be main-tained? It is within the crosshairs of these broader social concerns about healthcare, technology, and gender that hysterectomy patients find themselves. If the idea of terminating a single pregnancy incites such moral panic, I thought, what might it mean to willingly preclude the option of pregnancy by excising the uterus altogether?

Culture has the power to affect not only how medicine is provided but also how one feels about the medical experience. Researchers have found that people across cultures experience and understand biological symptoms differently—from menstruation,[12] to menopause,[13] to hormonal birth control[14]—in what the anthropologist Margaret Lock calls "local biologies." This led me to wonder: How might the stories we tell about hysterectomy, namely, that it's a negative experience or medical last resort, vary when you take a closer look through the eyes of those who want it?

This book does not tell a straightforwardly joyful, pro-hysterectomy story, even as I reject the assumption that the procedure is always terrible. The more one learns about hysterectomy, the more complicated the story becomes, both to the people who have (and don't succeed in having) the procedure and to the medical providers who perform (and don't perform) it. Tracing hysterectomy's historical roots, for instance, leads to chilling stories of medical experimentation, forced sterilizations, and eugenics. The staggering mortality and complication rates that accompanied early hysterectomies, and which largely deemed them the final plea of terminally ill women, underscore the complicated history of hysterectomy. Not to mention, hysterectomy continues to be performed disproportionately on Black, Indigenous, and other people of color, while alternatives to hysterectomy for managing chronic reproductive illness—some of which occur most frequently among women of color—are still far and few between.[15] These lines of inquiry speak to the darker side of gendered medical technology, in which hysterectomy is implicated.

Hysterectomy is also entangled in cultural and political battles within the highly contested sphere of trans rights. The World Professional Association for Transgender Health (WPATH) deems a hysterectomy an essential part of trans healthcare, and the science is unambiguous that accessing desired gender-affirming healthcare improves mental health and reduces suicide risk.[16] Hysterectomy has been a part of trans medicine since the early to mid-twentieth century, and the removal of the uterus has long been viewed as a gender-affirming procedure.[17] Yet the ability for trans and nonbinary people to access hysterectomy is caught in an ideological debate. The further trans health and inclusion make it into mainstream cultural conversations, the more vigorous anti-trans vitriol seems to become. Anti-trans legislation has been introduced in unprecedented numbers since 2021. In 2024, 45 of 665 proposed anti-trans bills have passed and been signed into law as I write this introduction, with 128 other proposed bills still active.[18] These anti-trans bills vary widely in severity, with the worst classifying gender-affirming care for kids as "child abuse" in Texas, Wyoming, and Minnesota.[19] As I examine who can choose a hysterectomy and why, taking a trans-inclusive approach reveals additional insight into how gender shapes all clinical encounters, as patients experience contradictory recommendations and barriers to care for the same procedure based on whether they are cis or trans.

Medical research has overlooked cis women's health and trans health like, leaving many questions unanswered with regard to reproductive and sexual health writ large as well as hysterectomy specifically, for people of all genders.[20] The constrained healthcare alternatives to hysterectomy, sparse biomedical research on illnesses of the uterus and ovaries, and a complicated sociopolitical and legal backdrop combined lead us to the question: What does it mean to *choose* hysterectomy? And, more critically, is it really *choosable* in a healthcare system that manages to both neglect and overmedicalize those with a uterus?

To explore my research questions, I collected and analyzed one hundred diverse hysterectomy stories from people who want, have had, or are considering an "elective" hysterectomy. These are not hysterectomies that are performed to avert death but rather the nine out of ten hysterectomies that are performed to treat chronic illness or as part of gender-affirming healthcare.[21] I recruited a sample of interviewees who varied in race and ethnicity, age, sexual orientation, and gender identity in order to capture a range of hysterectomy experiences, and the interviews took place over Zoom or on the phone. Participants in this study either had a chronic reproductive illness or identified as trans or nonbinary, and a small handful of interviewees fit into both categories. My sample was nearly evenly split between cisgender women and trans and/or nonbinary interviewees. I found participants primarily online, targeting social media pages organized around chronic reproductive issues or transgender interests and health. I also relied on snowball sampling, and various participants pointed me to friends or relatives. I also disseminated my digital recruitment flyer in listservs and online groups. (See the appendix for more information on my data collection and analysis.)

To be clear, while the medical system may determine these hysterectomies to be *elective*, participants do not. An insurance company might refuse to cover the cost of a hysterectomy, and one's provider and/or the hospital system might deem that procedure unnecessary. However, a hysterectomy is a treatment for a disease that renders one bedridden, in constant pain, gender dysphoric, or unable to have sex, making it for many anything but elective. While the uterus itself remains the same—a hollow, fist-sized, pear-shaped organ that lives in the pelvis—the way the body is externally racialized and gendered bestows distinct meanings on this particular part of the body. Looking closely at the various meanings deduced from these differently "housed" uteruses reveals the extent to which culture and politics interact with biological and structural forces to shape the experience of healthcare and of one's own body.

WHAT IS HYSTERECTOMY IN THE CONTEXT OF STRATIFIED REPRODUCTION?

Before we proceed, a basic epidemiological overview is needed. Hysterectomy can be either subtotal (the removal of the uterus only) or, more commonly, total (the removal of the uterus and the cervix). It can be accompanied by oophorectomy (the removal of one or both ovaries), a salpingectomy (removal of one or both fallopian tubes), or a salpingo-oophorectomy. Ovaries are often retained and fallopian tubes removed because while the former produce low levels of hormones throughout the lifespan and hence can be beneficial to overall health, the fallopian tubes are where many ovarian cancers originate.[22] In the case of a total hysterectomy, the top of the vaginal canal, which connects to the cervix, is sewed up into a vaginal "cuff." About a third of hysterectomies in the United States are performed alongside a bilateral oophorectomy, which leads to surgical menopause.[23] The occurrence of this type of hysterectomy is disproportionately higher among Black and Latine women.[24]

Hysterectomy is an identical procedure when performed on cis women or trans and nonbinary people; people of all genders typically have some say in which organs, other than the uterus itself, to keep or remove. Some trans and nonbinary people choose to keep their ovaries in order to have a production of hormones in case they one day lose access to pharmaceutically produced testosterone, since the body needs a source of hormones.[25]

A surgeon performs hysterectomies in a hospital setting either abdominally, laparoscopically, or hysteroscopically—procedures that are regarded, respectively, as most to least invasive. An abdominal hysterectomy entails a six- to twelve-inch cross-body incision, a procedure time of one to four hours followed by two to three days of hospitalization, and six to twelve weeks of recovery. Given the large cross-body incision it entails, abdominal hysterectomy is considered the most invasive and is associated with the greatest risks. A laparoscopic or robotic hysterectomy is considered minimally invasive and is performed through several small incisions on the abdomen; this type of surgery is typically outpatient or requires a single night of hospitalization and involves five incisions of twelve millimeters each, a procedure time of one to four hours, and a recovery time of two to six weeks. The least invasive approach, hysteroscopic vaginal hysterectomy, requires no abdominal incisions: the uterus is removed through a small incision at the top of the vagina in a procedure lasting one to four hours; hospitalization is one to two nights, and recovery time is three to four weeks.[26] Given hysterectomy's safety and its ability to address a variety of health concerns, most insurance plans cover hysterectomies deemed "medically necessary." However, as I will show throughout the book, "necessity" when it comes to diseases of the uterus and ovaries is highly subjective and socially constructed.

A patient fighting for a hysterectomy to improve their quality of life rather than turning to the procedure as the sole alternative to death would have been unimaginable until recent decades. As chapter 1 will detail, hysterectomy transformed over the centuries from one of the most brutal and risky medical procedures to one commonly referred to as "minimally invasive, outpatient surgery." I argue that the contemporary possibility of *choosing* an elective hysterectomy is driven by the surgical procedure's technical refinement—namely, the development of laparoscopic hysterectomy in 1988, when a large cross-abdominal incision and months of recovery were replaced with small "keyhole" incisions and a quick healing time. In a blog post titled "Not Your Mother's Hysterectomy," published on the website of a California-based obstetrician-gynecologist (ob-gyn) practice, the modern hysterectomy is described in the following way:

> Contemporary hysterectomies performed on an outpatient basis have become the norm. The procedure itself takes about an hour, and you'll be home the same day. Keyhole incisions produce little blood and the risk of complications stays low. If you need pain relief after your procedure, over-the-counter pain medications are usually up to the task, removing the need for opioid drugs. Your post-surgical downtime is typically 7 to 10 days. The tiny keyhole incisions mean that scars are equally tiny, if they form at all.[27]

New techniques for hysterectomy technologically transformed the procedure—making it safer, with a much shorter postoperative downtime, diminished pain, and minimal scarring. These transformations render hysterectomy more desirable and potentially more marketable. And yet, as chapter 3 will detail, while providers promote the vast improvements in and increased desirability of the modern hysterectomy, they continue to gatekeep access to it for patients they deem too young, not sick enough, or in need of protection from their own desires. As such, the modern hysterectomy is medically and technologically better than ever, and yet access to it is subject to the whims of providers, insurance companies, and hospital systems.

After cesarean sections, hysterectomy is the most common surgical procedure in the United States among people who are assigned female at birth (AFAB). While one out of ten hysterectomies is performed to treat cancer of the uterus, cervix, or ovaries, the remaining 90 percent are primarily understood to be "elective" procedures, meaning for purposes other than to save a life. The most common conditions associated with hysterectomy are uterine fibroids (which occur disproportionately among Black women),[28] uterine prolapse, and abnormal uterine bleeding, which could be due to endometriosis or adenomyosis.[29] Relative to the majority of Europe, Australia, and New Zealand, hysterectomy is three to four times more common in the United States, though rates differ by region and by race. Hysterectomy is more commonly performed on Black, Latine, and American Indian women, relative to non-Hispanic white women,[30] and it is performed at higher rates in the US South and Midwest, relative to other regions of the country. Throughout the book, I begin to unpack what might be leading to these different rates by disentangling the way social inequality impacts the unequal provision of hysterectomy.

Trans and nonbinary individuals are an often-overlooked population for whom hysterectomy is also common. For cis women, the vast majority of hysterectomies are deemed "elective." By contrast, a hysterectomy is considered an essential component of gender-affirming care for trans people and nonbinary people.[31] In fact, hysterectomy is the most common form of "bottom surgery" for trans men.[32] Approximately 14 to 21 percent of trans men have had a hysterectomy, while another 58 percent desire having one in the future. In regard to nonbinary AFAB people, only 2 percent have had a hysterectomy, though 30 percent want one. The prevailing reason for seeking a hysterectomy (58 percent) is the incongruence between their gender identity and having a uterus.[33] Additionally, 47 percent seek a hysterectomy as part of the process toward physical masculinization, 43 percent for legal documentation, and 37 percent to avert the need for ob-gyn care in the future (e.g., no more pap smears if you no longer have a vaginal canal or a cervix).

Given the myriad gaps in trans medical research,[34] agreement on the biological necessity of a hysterectomy to prevent reproductive cancers and other chronic issues for individuals undergoing hormone replacement therapy has not coalesced. It also remains unclear how difficult it is for trans and nonbinary people to access a hysterectomy, and how one feels afterward. This book digs into these unexplored questions within trans healthcare.

Findings regarding the impacts of a hysterectomy—both physiological and psychological—are mixed. Hysterectomy shares many of the risks inherent to other surgeries, including complications related to anesthesia, accidental damage to surrounding organs during surgery, infection, or blood clots. Additionally, because organs shift internally after hysterectomy, which can cause incontinence and other issues, the pelvic floor may need to be supported surgically, and post-operative pelvic floor therapy is critical. Some clinicians have concerns about posthysterectomy sexual functioning, as there are various nerve endings in the cervix—an organ that also provides some moisture during sex via cervical mucus. However, most people report unchanged or improved sex after hysterectomy—particularly if pain and bleeding were interfering with their sex lives.[35]

The uncontested effects of a hysterectomy are loss of menstruation, onset of (in some cases, early) menopause (even if the ovaries are retained), and loss of fertility (also called sterility). A person undergoing hysterectomy could theoretically preserve their fertility via egg or embryo freezing, but there are currently various barriers to access to such technologies in the United States, including lack of information and lack of insurance coverage and other financial burdens. Notably, medical egg freezing is rarely covered by private or state health insurance, while its coverage is mandatory in other nations.[36] Hence, in the case of hysterectomy, patients are often choosing between the benefits of the procedure—whether managing a chronic condition or as part of gender-affirming care—and their reproductive capability. This highlights how opting into hysterectomy can be viewed as choosing to be sterilized—a decision that is complicated by a history of forced sterilization based on gender, race, class, and disability.

Hysterectomy is also a story of *reproductive stratification*, whereby one's social positionality, particularly race, class, location, and citizenship, shapes one's ability to make reproductive choices.[37] Take the few explosive hysterectomy stories that have made international headlines in recent years. At the beginning of 2018, Lena Dunham, an actress, director, and producer, culminated her decade-long battle with endometriosis with a hysterectomy at the age of thirty-one.[38] Despite her wealth of resources—social and financial—this hysterectomy did not come easy to her. "I check myself into the hospital and announce I am not leaving until they stop this pain or take my uterus," she wrote in *Vogue*. "No, really, take her." Endometriosis can lead to fertility issues, including increased risk of miscarriage—which her doctors confirmed, yet they were reluctant to irreversibly remove this capacity surgically. "Their goal is to preserve my fertility," she writes. Dunham spent twelve days at the hospital until a hysterectomy was finally granted to her, and she documented this experience through Instagram selfies from her hospital bed and photos of her surgery scars. Dunham's story rippled into cultural conversations, sparking discussions about endometriosis and chronic pelvic pain and inspiring some, including some interviewees in this book, to start similar fights to have their own uteruses removed. Her story, while seldom told, is anything but unique and in fact is echoed by dozens of hysterectomy seekers in this book.

As a sharp contrast, only two years after Dunham's story, hysterectomy once more made international headlines. One account from NPR titled "Whistleblower Alleges 'Medical Neglect,' Questionable Hysterectomies of ICE Detainees" described women detained at a Georgia ICE facility who had been coerced into having hysterectomies without their fully informed consent, often due to language barriers.[39] Hysterectomies that are coercive in yet a different way are also expected to rise due to post-*Dobbs* abortion bans that prevent physicians from performing abortions, even if the pregnancy poses an immediate physical threat to life. In the summer of 2023, for instance, ProPublica reported the story of a Tennessee woman having an emergency hysterectomy after doctors refused to treat her ectopic pregnancy with abortion, as Tennessee is a state that punishes doctors who terminate a pregnancy with up to fifteen years of jail.[40] In a second term of a Trump presidency, with the possibility of a national abortion ban and further restrictions on abortion medications, coercive and emergency hysterectomies will likely increase.

Comparing these coercive hysterectomy stories with Dunham's *Vogue* feature reveals a continued tale of reproductive stratification. In one explosive hysterectomy story, an affluent white woman fights her doctors to have them remove her uterus, in defiance of what she perceives as their goal of preserving her fertility. In the other set of stories, women are stripped of their fertility and a vital organ at the hands of the state. As the chapters in this book will reveal, these few news stories are indicative of broader themes, in which the way one comes to have a hysterectomy largely hinges on who you are, where you live, and the resources at your disposal. What a hysterectomy means to you also reflects your historical and cultural relationship to stratified reproduction.

HYSTERECTOMY AS A TECHNOFIX

The modern hysterectomy is emblematic of a transformation of healthcare. Although medicine once referred to the treatment of disease, the current medical landscape expands far beyond these restricted uses. Medical providers are no longer tasked simply with identifying and alleviating illness but also with "transforming" and "fixing" bodies to fit social and cultural needs. Amid this transformation of healthcare—which sociologists refer to as *biomedicalization*—new biomedical technologies allow for bodily "customization," which improves one's quality of life, without necessarily saving it.[41] These technologies include cochlear implants, cosmetic surgeries, joint replacements, and assisted reproductive technologies like in vitro fertilization (IVF), all of which involve using biomedical tools to enhance the body and its processes. Rather than eradicating illness, these procedures allow individuals access to *socio-cultural* identities. By accessing them, each person has the chance to become someone or something else: a hearing person, a beautiful person, a walking person, a fertile person.

We are also flooded with and able to access health information—anyone can now google their symptoms, consult WebMD, or pull up articles from medical journals to arrive at a diagnosis or treatment plan. Subsequently, the notions of health risk and risk detection have become a normalized part of medicine. This relatively new calculus of "risk" compels all people to monitor and attempt to mitigate their own risks as well as undergo medical testing to identify risk. Think, for instance, of how prenatal testing has become an assumed norm, despite the uncertainty in its results.[42] In this system, then, "health" is not simply the absence of disease but rather an amorphous, perpetually out of reach category to which we all constantly aspire. We have all the tools at our disposal—technological and knowledge based—to seek to be as "healthy" as possible. We can monitor our caloric intake, identify and reduce carcinogenic exposures, and track our heartbeats and our steps on iPhones. We pour thousands of dollars into preventative medicine and procedures of enhancement and optimization, as opposed to treatments and cures. Health, then, is both a status symbol and a moralized pursuit.[43] To engage in and embody "unhealthy" behaviors, including having a chronic illness that interferes with your life, then, symbolically denotes some sort of moral failure against this cultural backdrop.

It is in this biomedicalized world that an elective hysterectomy is situated, as hysterectomy can be used to customize the body, forge a new identity, or improve one's quality of life. Many people who recount their experiences in this book describe their hysterectomy as a tool to fix a "broken or erroneous body" or to remove a "pesky organ" that is causing problems. At the same time, a hysterectomy can be lifesaving, or profoundly life enhancing, whether or not modern medicine or insurance plans regard it as such. For many, excising one's uterus opens up a world in which schedules and mental well-being do not hinge on the whims of their body; where they can plan a vacation or pursue an education or a career without worrying about the symptoms brought on by their uterus. You might not die from being bound to your couch from extreme pain or from the gender dysphoria brought on by menstruation, but your mental health and quality of life will certainly suffer. Hence, as chapter 2 will detail, many view hysterectomy as a "tool in the toolbox," which grants new possibilities in how they experience their body and move through the world.

Given the benefits of hysterectomy to many, there is a fundamental contradiction in the way its provision is variously controlled and encouraged. Hysterectomy patients live in a culture that compels them to be as "healthy" as possible, to acquire as much knowledge about their body, and to use every tool at their disposal. Yet that very culture—the individuals and systems of power that constitute it—can still block them from the freedom to *choose* this tool. The ability to use technoscience to forge new identities or to "fix" an imperfect or broken body is constrained or enhanced by social privilege.

One's access to a hysterectomy is also caught up in powerful cultural narratives that impact medicine—specifically, stereotypes about the "female body," race, pain, and trans identities. Simply obtaining a diagnosis for certain conditions that can lead to a hysterectomy, such as endometriosis, adenomyosis, or fibroids, can be exceedingly difficult. The arduous path to diagnosis for these illnesses is rooted in cultural ideas about women's pain, which are only magnified by racial stereotypes for women of color, given the demonstrated link between race and the minimization of pain, particularly among Black patients.[44] Researchers attribute these wait times to the normalization of pelvic pain as "normal period pain" that individuals must overcome by changing their health behaviors (e.g., by losing weight, changing exercise and diet).[45] Rigid cultural ideas around gender also come to bear in hysterectomy for trans health, as providers can gatekeep access through a specific set of requirements to prove one's transness or need for surgery.[46] Additionally, "women's bodies" are largely treated as one-day pregnant—or, in other words, *at risk* of pregnancy—starting from puberty, in a way that shapes the care and medical advice women and girls receive by ushering them toward fertility retention.[47] These culturally specific notions of bodies—bodies in pain, bodies that must adhere to a sex and gender binary, bodies that must one day be pregnant—can lead to long delays to hysterectomy or to it never being uttered as an option.

Despite various barriers to care, patients have long mobilized to effect change within medicine. From feminist efforts to change standards of care for ob-gyn and breast cancer,[48] to the HIV/AIDS social movement in the 1980s and 1990s,[49] women, communities of color, and gender and sexual minorities have historically challenged the healthcare system. This collective action shapes public knowledge and draws attention to previously ignored medical needs and abuses. This dynamic continues in the present day as groups mobilize around "women's issues" such as fibromyalgia,[50] endometriosis,[51] obstetric violence and racism,[52] or pressure to use contraceptive technologies even in the face of side effects.[53] The hysterectomy stories in this book show a continuation of these collective efforts. In the process of seeking a hysterectomy, many are challenging and rebuilding a healthcare system that has not been designed with their needs in mind.

REPRODUCTIVE JUSTICE AND (IN)FERTILITY

In response to the limitations of a "reproductive rights" framework—which often focuses on the right to abortion and contraception—the Black Women's Caucus in the 1990s coined *reproductive justice* to conceptualize the universal right to all reproductive, bodily, and sexual autonomy.[54] Reproductive justice is a framework with three primary principles: that all people have (1) the right not to have a child, (2) the right to have a child, and (3) the right to raise children in safe and healthy environments. In addition, reproductive justice demands sexual autonomy and gender freedom for every human being.[55] The diverse set of hysterectomy interviews I draw from reveals the various ways reproductive justice can be violated, as well as the multiple mechanisms of eugenics logic. As I argue throughout this book, preventing some people from being able to actively choose a hysterectomy and coercing others into having a hysterectomy are both forms of reproductive injustice.[56] Moreover, the stratified choice of a hysterectomy fits within what the sociologist and legal scholar Dorothy Roberts and others reference as positive or negative eugenics.[57] *Positive eugenics* refers to "improving the race" through encouragement of some births, while *negative eugenics* refers to eliminating "socially inadequate" births. Unequal access to a hysterectomy continues this legacy by preserving socially adequate fertility and coercively removing socially inadequate fertility. Amid this stratification, the ability to make informed health decisions and thus live self-determined lives is restricted for all people with uteruses, albeit in differently gendered and racialized ways.

Hysterectomy is inextricably linked to reproductive justice as it produces an infertile or sterilized body and identity. Work examining the intersections of technology and infertility focuses on two primary areas of inquiry: using biomedicine to *overcome* infertility and using biomedicine to force sterility upon people through state-sanctioned sterilization abuse. In both cases, infertility is nonconsensual and is thus largely discussed as a ruinous experience, for instance, centering the isolation, grief, and feelings of worthlessness felt by infertile women.[58] There has been less work examining how infertility is jointly constructed by these two discourses—on a continuum between choice and constraint and shaped by gendered and racialized processes in tandem. Moreover, while infertility research tends to center the experience of cis, heterosexual women, I explicitly include hysterectomy stories from queer and trans people, groups that have negotiated reproductive healthcare to forge queer reproduction despite broader pushback to queer families. The hysterectomy stories in this book expose the often-blurred boundary between choice and constraint within reproductive healthcare, especially for women of color, queer and trans populations, and those who don't fit the image of "ideal reproducer."

ORGANIZATION OF THE BOOK

As I will aim to make clear in the following chapters, hysterectomy provides a robust case for understanding the complicated relationships between medicine, gender, race, reproduction, and technology. Chapter 1, "How Hysterectomy's History Shapes Its Present," contextualizes modern hysterectomy stories within the history of medicine, specifically within three major legacies of modern medicine: (1) the emergence of medicine to treat "women's disorders," (2) racialized medical abuse and experimentation, and (3) the development of transgender healthcare. Throughout this chapter, I show how modern hysterectomy experiences are shaped by the legacies of medical sexism (including the hegemony of hysteria and medical experimentation on women's bodies), eugenics movements and forced sterilization, and the development of trans medicine in the early twentieth century. By tracing these histories, this chapter demonstrates the ways in which present-day hysterectomy trends are largely examples of history repeating itself.

In chapters 2 through 5, I center the voices of the people I interviewed—the true "experts" in this research. Chapter 2, "Why Would Someone Want a Hysterectomy?," examines the reclaiming of hysterectomy from an "unnecessary," overperformed instrument of an oppressive healthcare system to a tool individuals can use to "fix" or enhance a broken or erroneous body. In the process, I interrogate how in a medical system ill-equipped to treat the various illnesses and conditions associated with the uterus and ovaries, hysterectomy becomes a desired procedure. In chapter 3, "Who Can 'Choose' Hysterectomy?," I examine how one's ability to choose a hysterectomy is limited by a constellation of reproductive politics and stratified reproduction. Race and gender largely shape medical recommendations for the same procedure, as clinicians, hospital systems, and insurance companies unequally gatekeep or encourage access to hysterectomy for seemingly social, rather than strictly medical, reasons.

Chapter 4, "How Do People Feel about Hysterectomy?," interrogates the common clinician assumption that one will come to regret a hysterectomy by investigating the various reactions people have about this surgery. In particular, this chapter unpacks how the reproductive politics that stratify access to hysterectomy also stratify the various reactions to the surgery—from grief to delight to somewhere in between. Chapter 5, "Navigating Access to Hysterectomy," uncovers the ways hysterectomy seekers must rely on alternative sources of knowledge, community networks, and social media, as well as social and cultural health capital, to achieve their health goals.[59] Amid health inequity, strategies to challenge the medical system—by becoming a "rowdy patient"—prove critical to the ability to make health choices.

I conclude by connecting these one hundred hysterectomy stories to the ongoing struggles for reproductive, sexual, and gender freedom that extend much further than the surgical excision of the uterus. The stories in this book not only demonstrate the resilience and strength of these patients and their communities but also call for a better world—one that values uteruses and the people who have them; one that invests in researching, understanding, and healing these gendered organs; and one where healthcare is accessible, trans competent, and aligned with the values of reproductive justice.

1

HOW HYSTERECTOMY'S HISTORY SHAPES ITS PRESENT

> Now one must not suppose the uterus to be essential to life. For not only does it prolapse, but in some cases . . . it has even been cut away without bringing death.
> —Soranus of Ephesus

Hysterectomy has been around for millennia, but there are a few discrete threads in this procedure's long, winding history that help explain the inequalities we see in its provision today. Hysterectomy has played key roles in three critical epochs in medical history: in the treatment of "women's maladies" from the time of hysteria onward, as part of state-sanctioned sterilization and eugenics projects, and as an element of the formation of trans healthcare in the twentieth century. Tracing these interrelated histories is key to understanding present-day hysterectomy narratives. In the process, trying to understand hysterectomy's history ends up unfurling the way the creation of medicine—including the formation of gynecology and trans health—is inextricable from a legacy of sexism, racism, slavery, and colonialism. Going back to where it all began will help us understand how we got here—how hysterectomy at its core is unchoosable, stratified, and burdened by history.

THE BIRTH OF HYSTERECTOMY: WOMEN'S MALADIES AND WANDERING WOMBS

Though we think of surgery as a modern medical marvel, the earliest hysterectomies are believed to have been performed in ancient Greece by Themison of Athens in 50 BC and by Soranus of Ephesus in AD 120.[1] These early procedures were vaginal hysterectomies—meaning the uterus is removed through an incision at the top of the vagina at the cervix—and were mostly done to resolve physical ailments such as a prolapsed uterus, fibroids, or ovarian tumors. Women rarely survived. Despite their extreme danger, there are records of these early hysterectomies being performed by healers throughout the Middle Ages.[2] There is also lore of midwives performing hysterectomies for patients and one particularly striking story of a peasant woman performing the operation on herself in 1670.[3] While hard to believe, this case was well documented and, alongside the history of midwives performing hysterectomies, points to a long-standing historical legacy of women taking control of their own reproductive healthcare. At the same time, these highly dangerous, experimental surgeries took place in a world without medical alternatives, and without adequate research into the conditions necessitating them. In the twenty-first century, little has changed in this regard.

What *has* changed is the immense technological refinement of surgery: we now have a concept of a "minimally invasive surgery" and specifically of a minimally invasive hysterectomy. Surgical advancements, it turns out, are rooted in experimentation on the bodies of women. The first recorded abdominal surgery was performed to remove a twenty-two-pound ovarian cyst on a woman named Jane Crawford by Dr. Ephraim McDowell in Kentucky in 1809. Rather than accept the death sentence that an ovarian cyst would have typically been at that time, Jane agreed to undergo this very first procedure of its kind before the advent of anesthesia or antisepsis—instead, she sang hymns throughout the surgery to endure the pain.[4] Despite its seeming impossibility, both at the time and in retrospect, Jane survived the surgery, and many now regard McDowell as the "father of modern surgery." The Ephraim McDowell House in Danville, Kentucky, erected to commemorate McDowell, credits this particular surgery on Jane with paving the way for modern surgery.[5] After this milestone, surgery's refinement sped up as experimentation on women with illnesses continued to flourish.

As Christopher Sutton, a professor of gynecological surgery, writes in a 1997 historical account: "Early records of the first abdominal hysterectomies read like a disaster saga."[6] These early days of abdominal hysterectomies—abjectly horrific for the women, yet instrumental social spectacles for the physicians—occurred before three key developments that we now consider essential to surgery: the widespread use of anesthesia in surgery beginning in 1846, the rise of antiseptic surgery from 1876, and the clinical use of antibiotics starting in the

1940s. For years, these early hysterectomies were overwhelmingly fatal: both their exploratory nature and the lack of surgical advancements mentioned previously led to frequent physician-caused major complications (e.g. by accidentally removing the bladder or ureter during a surgery). Patients often died of infection, hemorrhage, or exhaustion. The first person to have an abdominal hysterectomy, performed by Dr. Charles Clay in Manchester, England, in 1843, died fifteen days after the procedure after falling out of bed. The mortality risk for these procedures was around 70 percent even as late as the 1880s, and they were regarded as a last resort for ill women without alternatives, with doctors only performing hysterectomies on women who had terminal reproductive conditions.[7]

In the Age of Heroic Medicine, between 1780 and 1850, when medical practices were characterized by rigorous and extreme procedures to shock the body back to health, it was commonplace for surgeons to invite other men, medical colleagues and nonmedical friends, to witness, unmasked and ungloved, medical events such as these early hysterectomies. During this time, some doctors chose to perform surgery without anesthesia even after it became relatively standard; for instance, Dr. Clay felt that anesthesia "interfered with his good results," as only patients willing to endure the surgery without it had the will to survive, as Sutton recounts.[8] Many medical historians believe early gynecology, which, along with obstetrics, emerged as a field at the end of the nineteenth century, was at the forefront of the professionalization of modern medicine.[9] Without this rampant experimentation on women's bodies, then, modern medicine as we know it would not have coalesced.[10]

As the stories in this book will show, many decision-wielding figures within healthcare—physicians, hospital policymakers, and insurance companies—continue to regard hysterectomy as a "last resort," despite the immense technological advancements and improved safety in the procedure. Today's hysterectomy is nearly unrecognizable from these early forms, due primarily to the development of lap-

aroscopic hysterectomy in 1988 by Dr. Harry Reich in Pennsylvania.
Hysterectomy is now regarded as a safe, highly common surgery used
to address a variety of health concerns.[11] And yet, the pervasive belief
about hysterectomy's dangers can lead to restricted access even for
those who want it.

HYSTERICAL WOMBS AND HYSTERECTOMY

Examining hysterectomies requires delving into the history of *hysteria*—a broadly nebulous term for a mysterious disease whereby
any issue a woman might be experiencing could be blamed on her
uterus. Hysterectomy and hysteria, as some readers may have noticed,
are connected through the shared Greek etymological root *hystera*,
or "womb." From the time of Hippocrates in ancient Greece up
until the 1950s, it was a common belief across cultures that a slew
of women's ailments and problems—social and biological, real and
illusory—were due to a "wandering womb." The disease of hysteria,
it was believed, indicated a uterus on the loose that roamed the body
searching for unborn babies, wreaking havoc in its path and causing
any of a multitude of symptoms.[12] Hysteria translates both to "womb
disease" and to "woman's disease," as well as to "suffocation of the
mother" and "suffocation of the womb."[13] This medical language in
history points to a long-standing conflation of woman with womb,
which continues on in the present day in the medical framing of all
women as one-day mothers.[14] So, in addition to sharing the Greek
root meaning both "uterus" and "woman," the terms *hysterectomy*
and *hysteria* also share roots in the same age-old gendered notion:
that anything which troubles women—physically, psychologically, or
socially—must be caused by the presence of the uterus, the organ
long believed to separate women from men.

While hysteria as a paradigm of illness was persistent across time
and geographic location, it is nearly impossible to neatly define.
Instead, hysteria amounted to what the historian Edward Shorter

calls "a blizzard of symptoms" that adapted to "the ideas and mores current in each society."[15] However vague, symptoms of hysteria generally included nervousness, irritability, anxiety, insomnia, unexplained pain, irregular menstrual bleeding, and fainting. Other symptoms included "erotic fantasy, sensations of heaviness in the abdomen, lower pelvic edema, and vaginal lubrication"—symptoms that, as the historian Rachel Maines notes in her book *The Technology of Orgasm: "Hysteria," the Vibrator, and Women's Sexual Satisfaction*, are indications of normal female sexual arousal.[16] Given the wide variation in symptoms, historians agree that hysteria was ultimately used as a catchall term to pathologize not only physical and psychological symptoms but also cultural and social deviations from feminine gender norms, anything from "excessive sexuality" to childlessness (hence the uterus's search for unborn babies) to lack of interest in sex.[17] Perhaps most notably, hysteria was rooted in a belief in uterine dominance: the idea that women's behaviors are heavily influenced, if not controlled, by the uterus. It therefore follows that among the many documented physician recommendations for hysteria—including clitorectomies, physician-performed massages to orgasm, and herbs—hysterectomy was used to treat this malady exclusive to women.[18]

The American Psychiatric Association officially dropped the term *hysteria* along with no fewer than 250 "hystero-neurasthenic disorders" (*neurasthenia* being a blanket term for weakness of the nerves) from the canon of modern disease paradigms in 1952. However, many scholars believe that the "hysterization of women's bodies," aptly named by the philosopher Michel Foucault,[19] has since been sustained by other realms of the medical-industrial complex. The feminist critic Elaine Showalter, in her book *Hystories: Hysterical Epidemics and Modern Media*, argues that the sweeping psychiatric diagnosis of hysteria was replaced by a number of distinct modern illnesses implicitly associated with women, such as borderline personality disorder, histrionic personality disorder, and depression.[20]

Three-quarters of borderline personality disorder diagnoses today are given to women; moreover, women are four times more likely than men to be diagnosed with histrionic personality disorder and twice as likely to be diagnosed with depression, the most common mental disorder in the United States.[21] These disparities are partially driven by gendered stereotypes of women as overly emotional or dramatic—a belief that has long reduced the quality of healthcare women receive and continues in present-day healthcare provision, as experienced by hysterectomy seekers in this book.

In addition to hysteria's frequent insinuation into psychiatric illnesses, the legacy of hysteria also endures in various diseases associated with women's bodies, for which a hysterectomy is often indicated. In modern disease paradigms, much like hysteria, the illnesses and conditions that are associated with women—from PMS to fibromyalgia to fibroids—are largely thought of as mysterious or unknowable, incurable, and, perhaps most important, the consequence of a person failing to adhere to gendered expectations. The symptoms of these illnesses are often dismissed, ignored, or misdiagnosed because when it comes to pain, women are caught in a double bind. Women's pain is at once viewed as illusory, overdramatized, and a sign of neuroticism yet simultaneously as an inherent part of having a woman's body—or, as the feminist cultural critic Ella Shohat put it, bound up with the "melancholic fate of being a woman."[22]

Nowhere is this legacy of hysteria in "women's healthcare" more evident, however, than in endometriosis, an illness that often leads people to a hysterectomy. Endometriosis causes extreme pain and inflammation due to tissues similar to the uterine lining growing elsewhere in the body. Despite endometriosis growths being merely *similar* to the tissue found in the uterus, they are often described as uterine lining that wanders or roams, spreading and attaching itself throughout the body. For instance, *Yale Medicine* defines endometriosis as "when the normal lining of the uterus starts to grow outside the uterine wall," evoking an image of an uncontained, free-floating

uterine lining.[23] Also echoing the medical framing of hysteria, endometriosis is often discussed as mysterious and enigmatic, as well as
linked to childlessness and cured by pregnancy. There is no evidence
that pregnancy is a permanent cure, though some symptoms can
abate during the pregnancy, yet providers continue to recommend
pregnancy, including to people whose experiences are recounted in
this book.[24] Even medical textbooks long referred to endometriosis as
"the career woman's disease" and identified purportedly unfeminine
behaviors such as delaying childbearing as a cause of this illness.[25]
Endometriosis is therefore on the long list of "women's diseases" that
are influenced by and perpetuate beliefs about women and motherhood, and that continue to carry the torch of hysteria's past.

From what is now abundantly clear within the archives of medical
journals, many of the symptoms once attributed to hysteria are today's telltale endometriosis symptoms. For instance, in 1951, a group
of psychiatrists published an article titled "Observations on Clinical
Aspects of Hysteria" in the prestigious *Journal of the American Medical Association* in order to advance a consistent clinical picture of hysteria, which the authors acknowledged had previously been missing.
In their analysis, they write:

> Especially prominent symptoms were pain, menstrual difficulties,
> alleged difficulty during pregnancy and difficulty in sexual adjust-
> ment. . . . Not only was there a high frequency of symptoms in women
> with hysteria associated with menstrual, sexual and reproductive
> functions, but also were such symptoms described by the patients in a
> characteristic, colorful and dramatic fashion.[26]

I encourage readers to keep this description of hysterical women in
mind when reading the present-day accounts of people with chronic
reproductive illness, including endometriosis. These are certainly
stories that are "colorful and dramatic": stories of immense bleeding
through several layers of menstrual products and clothes, of being

unable to leave one's bed because of the pain, or of fainting in the middle of the workday. How many of these women would have been labeled hysterical a few decades ago or, worse, institutionalized, as were many women before them? How many of them were told they were exaggerating for years, until a doctor finally found the source of their agony?

HYSTERECTOMY AT THE HANDS OF THE STATE: EXPERIMENTATION AND STERILIZATION

Understanding contemporary hysterectomy patterns, perceptions, and experiences also requires an examination of race and racism throughout the development of "women's healthcare." In fact, any historical account of women's healthcare would be decidedly incomplete without examining how gynecology—and the medical-industrial complex writ large—was built on the experimentation and abuse of communities of color. Beginning with the antebellum South, Black women's bodies were essential to the economics of slavery, as slave owners had economic stakes in their reproduction. This led to collaborations between physicians and slaveowners to promote and preserve the fertility of women living in slavery. Many of the (white) women I mentioned previously who underwent early experimental hysterectomies agreed to these procedures. While these choices were certainly constrained—no woman had full rights during this time— Black women living under slavery did not have any degree of choice in having their bodies experimented upon. And yet, the refinement of the tools and techniques of the medical-industrial complex, including the tools and techniques of hysterectomy, is rooted in these inhumane, racialized experimentations.

One doctor in particular, Dr. J. Marion Sims, has become the face of the egregious, racialized history of gynecology in the United States. Examining his legacy helps explain not only the reproductive stratification of today's hysterectomies but also how patients of color make sense of their hysterectomy experiences. Sims practiced medicine in Alabama from 1835 until his death in the early 1880s, during which time he came to be regarded as the "father of gynecology." He is particularly known for the development of the duckbill speculum, still referred to by some, albeit controversially, as the Sims speculum—including by the International Planned Parenthood Federation in its *Client-Centred Clinical Guidelines for Sexual and Reproduction Healthcare* (2022) and in the permanent installation of the Sex Museum in New York City.[27] Sims developed this speculum, and his various other gynecological achievements, after a yearslong series of horrific experimental surgeries on three enslaved women, Betsey, Anarcha, and Lucy. These three women are now often referred to as the "mothers of gynecology," a deserved reassignment of Sims's title. When interacting with medical providers, including while choosing a hysterectomy, many patients today must grapple with how the field of gynecology originated in, and continues to be haunted by, slavery and exploitation.

Hysterectomy is also entangled in histories of race science and eugenics, which proliferated long after slavery was abolished in the United States in 1865. In 1907, the first US eugenics law was passed in Indiana, allowing for the forced sterilization of "confirmed criminals, idiots, imbeciles, and rapists."[28] While Indiana's law initially targeted predominantly poor white men viewed as "hypersexual," including those suspected of "homosexuality," these laws soon came to target mainly poor women of color. Over the next two decades, thirty-two US states established official forced sterilization programs or formal eugenics boards composed of physicians and government officials like state attorneys general or state directors of public health. In 1927, these programs were solidified by federal law and ruled constitutional by the Supreme Court in *Buck v. Bell*. In Justice Oliver Wendell Holmes's majority (8–1) opinion, he justified the use of forced sterilization as part of public welfare, as "society can prevent those who are manifestly unfit from continuing their kind."[29] *Buck v. Bell* was never formally overturned, though by the late 1970s most states had overturned their sterilization laws.

Choosing a hysterectomy today, given that it is a sterilization procedure, invokes these decades of forced sterilization at the hands of the state. Women, the poor, immigrants, and people of color, particularly Black women and girls, were disproportionately the victims of forced sterilization in the twentieth century, during which more than seventy thousand Americans were forcibly sterilized. In North Carolina alone—a state with one of the most aggressive eugenics programs—approximately seventy-six hundred people were forcibly sterilized during the program's fifty years of operation until it was disbanded in 1977. California, another state infamous for its role in the American eugenics movement and the third state to pass a eugenics law, forcibly sterilized around twenty thousand individuals in state institutions between 1909 and 1979.[30] As an aside, California's eugenics laws inspired Adolf Hitler's plans for ethnic cleansing in Europe, and there was regular communication between Hitler's administration and Californian eugenicists.[31] While on paper these sterilization policies targeted anyone deemed "feeble minded," "delinquent," dependent on welfare, or "promiscuous," gender and race were embedded in these definitions. As the historian Alexandra Minna Stern argues in her book *Eugenic Nation: Faults and Frontiers of Better Breeding in Modern America*, race was entrenched in definitions of "feeble-mindedness" and delinquency, and gender was interrogated through concerns about sexuality, fertility, and the right and the wrong way to be a parent—including pregnancy out of wedlock and parenting while in poverty.[32]

While poor Black women were the primary victims of forced sterilization programs, historians have traced the way racist stereotypes were weaponized against various communities of color who must also grapple with this history when considering a hysterectomy. The epidemiologist Nicole Novak and her team found that forced sterilization laws in California, for instance, were disproportionately wielded against Latine residents—particularly those of Mexican origin or Chicana women and girls.[33] Undergirding these racialized patterns lie racist beliefs about Mexican women's "hyper-fertility," promiscuity, and genetic inferiority.[34] Moreover, in 1976, the US Department of Health, Education, and Welfare reported that over 37 percent of women of childbearing age in Puerto Rico had been sterilized between the 1930s and the 1970s, a population whose high birth rates were of concern to US eugenicists.[35]

Rates of coerced and involuntary sterilization of Native women also rose in the late 1960s through the mid-1970s and remain high today. Many experts view these practices as both an extension of state-sponsored genocide and a continuation of the historical forced removal of Native children and subsequent adoption by non-Native families.[36] Around one of four Native American women during the 1970s alone are believed to have been sterilized through coercion, deception, or force, which includes reports of women being deceptively told that sterilizations could be reversed via tubes being untied or uteruses replaced through transplants.[37] In 1976, a study conducted by the US General Accounting Office found that between 1973 and 1976, four of the twelve Indian Health Service regions sterilized 3,406 Native American women without their permission, including three dozen who were under twenty-one.[38] Choosing hysterectomy, then, given the history of forced sterilization across racialized groups, takes on different meanings for various communities of color, for whom this "choice" was once a weapon of state-sanctioned racialized violence.

BIRTH CONTROL IN THE SHADOW OF EUGENICS

A race analysis of the development of birth control also helps explain the continued racial stratification in gynecology, which still haunts present-day hysterectomies. While US eugenics programs flourished, the nation was simultaneously concerned about white women's declining fertility as abortion and birth control gradually became mainstream throughout the twentieth century.[39] In an attempt to temper the rise of fertility-limiting technologies for white women, for instance, the Comstock Act was weaponized against birth control advocates and providers, including Margaret Sanger, a nurse and the founder of Planned Parenthood, who was arrested in 1916 for her work distributing contraceptives. Practices such as these, which seek to promote the fertility of white middle-class people, comprise "positive" eugenics, which refers to the encouragement of "good reproduction." This facet of eugenics is far less discussed, yet it is part and parcel of *stratified reproduction*, a term that captures how reproductive autonomy is structured across demographic, social, and cultural boundaries. Examining these twin problems of "positive" and "negative" eugenics in history helps frame the hysterectomy stories in this book.

Technologies that limit or remove one's fertility, like hysterectomy, can be viewed by some as empowering, and by others as tools of oppression. Considering how an oral hormonal contraceptive, or "the Pill," was developed helps explain these different perceptions. The Pill was approved by the FDA in 1960, a landmark moment that is widely considered a catalyst of the "sexual revolution." Yet the push to develop and distribute new and effective methods of birth control like the Pill was motivated by eugenicist desires for "population control" among nonwhite and poor populations.[40] Birth control as we know it today was in fact developed through exploitative and unethical experimentation on these very communities. In the 1950s, clinical trials for an oral hormonal contraceptive (produced under the brand name Enovid by G. D. Searle and Company), were conducted by Harvard professors in Puerto Rico; around fifteen hundred women took these pills, usually without being told of their potential side effects or even that they were intended to prevent pregnancy. The historian Laura Briggs writes that these trials "epitomize the way in which science subjected vulnerable women of Third World countries to dangerous side effects in order to develop a drug for middle-class White women."[41] In other words, the history of the Pill's development was simultaneously a history of violence for racialized women and a history of empowerment for middle-class white women. Given these divergent historical memories, how might a hysterectomy likewise be understood differently across racial and ethnic lines?

Following the Pill's overwhelmingly robust public reception, researchers began multiple additional Puerto Rico–based trials—for Depo-Provera (a hormonal contraceptive injection), spermicidal contraceptive foam, and the IUD—which are also now widely regarded as unethical, dangerous, and conducted largely without participants' informed consent.[42] On the mainland, a clinical trial for Depo-Provera was conducted in Atlanta between 1967 and 1978; 11,400 mostly poor Black women were the participants in this trial, during which serious side effects—including heavy bleeding and suicidal ideation—were documented. These histories help explain the high levels of medical mistrust among Black, Latine, and Native patients we still see today.[43] Black and Latine women, for instance, are more likely to believe the government presently uses women of color and the poor to test birth control and that birth control is used to limit minority populations.[44] Choosing a procedure like hysterectomy, then, which permanently removes one's ability for pregnancy, evokes different, racialized meanings rooted in this historical violence. These divergent histories help explain why a white woman might beg her doctor for a hysterectomy, whereas a Black, Latine, or Native woman might reject a doctor's recommendation for a hysterectomy.

Though the health literature often refers to medical mistrust as "conspiracy beliefs," this mistrust is not only accurately grounded in history but also reflected by present-day reproductive injustices within which hysterectomy is situated. As recently as May 2019, a Tennessee judge and county sheriff shortened people's jail sentences if they agreed to undergo vasectomy or a birth control implant—a choice that a federal court ruled coercive and unconstitutional.[45]

On the other side of the country, 150 women in California prisons were coerced into sterilizations between the years 2006 and 2010.[46] While the particular technology utilized in these sterilizations varies, hysterectomies specifically made headlines in the summer of 2020. A whistleblower at a US Immigration and Customs Enforcement (ICE) facility in Georgia alleged that forced and coerced hysterectomies were widely performed on detained migrant women, many of whom could not consent to the procedure, by a physician allegedly nicknamed the "Uterus Collector."[47] In a neighboring state, hysterectomies are so widespread for Black women, they have long been nicknamed "Mississippi appendectomies."[48]

Meanwhile, the promotion of births among white and high-income women also continues to shape healthcare provision. This orientation toward white middle-class births is evident in healthcare's investment in fertility treatments such as IVF, which is disproportionately financially feasible for white couples. The overturning of *Roe v. Wade* and the consequent spread of abortion bans can also be understood in this light of promotion of "good births." At the same time, Black, Indigenous, and Latine women are often encouraged or coerced to "choose" long-acting reversible contraceptives (LARCs), including the IUD, Depo-Provera, and hormonal contraceptive implants such as Norplant, due to being construed as "high-risk" within medicine for unwanted pregnancy.[49] As part of this racialized divergence in fertility promotion versus limitation, Medicaid covers various forms of contraception but not fertility treatments—and some insurance plans cover LARC insertion but not removal.[50] The hysterectomy stories in this book help illuminate these divergent promotions or fertility-enhancing or fertility-limiting technologies throughout history, as some people are encouraged toward the removal of their uterus while others are denied access to this surgery.

To truly understand the hysterectomy stories in this book, then, requires an intersectional, justice-oriented look that is grounded by a history of positive and negative eugenics policies and practices. This requires one to grapple with the ways in which race and gender inequality concurrently shape these stories, and how these systems of oppression in tandem constrain one's ability to choose. At the same time, these histories are not destiny, and while hysterectomy has been differently weaponized, it is not inherently good or bad as a procedure in and of itself. Decisions about hysterectomy, like all elements of reproductive health, cannot be adequately captured in simplistic or binary terms alone but rather should be seen as operating on a continuum between coercion and choice, and as a refraction point between past and present.

HYSTERECTOMY AND THE ORIGINS OF TRANS HEALTH

Tracing the arc of trans medicine—its starts and stops, waves of progress followed by backlash—helps contextualize today's hysterectomy for trans and nonbinary patients. Though trans medicine is often framed in the media as a brand-new trend, it's actually older than antibiotics. Examining trans history alongside the history of gynecology and its racist, eugenicist origins sheds additional insight into how trans medicine came to be, as well as how deeply rooted stratified reproduction is within healthcare. Gynecology and surgery were developed via experimentation on cis women's bodies, refined via the exploitation of Black and brown women, and subsequently fashioned into what is now understood as trans medicine.[51] These histories have unfolded in tandem, underscoring the need for a trans-inclusive analysis of modern-day hysterectomy stories—and of all reproductive healthcare writ large.

Presently, all elements of trans health, including hysterectomy, are underresearched and underresourced, and trans competent care has yet to be fully integrated into medicine. Yet the first professionalized clinic devoted to trans health—referred to at the time as care for "sex intermediaires"—is more than one hundred years old.[52] The history of trans identities is even older. There is an extensive, established history of gender nonconformity and transness predating US colonial times, and before many had the language with which to name it. Trans historians have traced gender variability among various Indigenous societies, including in the written records of European colonizers in the Americas as early as the 1530s. The anthropologist Sabine Lang analyzed the recordings of conquistadors, missionaries, and traders for descriptions of gender variability, which she argues has been largely conflated with homosexuality through a moralized Western, Christian lens.[53]

There is also an extensive record of individuals in Western, postcolonial contexts dressing and living in a cross-gender manner, often in secret. The historian Susan Stryker, in her book *Transgender History: The Roots of Today's Revolution*, writes, "People who contradicted social expectations of what was considered typical for men or for women have existed since the earliest days of colonial settlement."[54] The various cross-dressing laws in the United States, dating back to the 1690s in Massachusetts, point to the presence of gender variation in this time and to a perceived social need to contain it. Additionally, the trans historian Jules Gill-Peterson recounts one hundred years of historical documentation of trans children in her book *Histories of the Transgender Child*. Many of these children successfully socially transitioned and subsequently medically transitioned once medical procedures were available in the mid-twentieth century.[55]

All in all, there are extensive records of trans existence across cultures and spanning several centuries, underscoring the illegitimacy of claims that being trans is a fleeting twenty-first-century trend that can be stopped by restrictive policies. The need for gender-affirming care, including hysterectomy, is therefore an integral part of modern medicine. The failure to properly integrate trans healthcare into "mainstream medicine," including investing in understanding trans hysterectomies, represents a failure rooted in social stigma rather than lack of long-standing determined need.

TREATING GENDER AND SEX IN THE CLINIC

Much as in gynecological care for women, the history of trans medicine helps explain present-day inequalities in healthcare, including in the provision of hysterectomy. While gender diversity in a social capacity had long existed, it entered the medical sphere at the turn of the twentieth century. Tracing the momentum toward developing gender-affirming healthcare, followed by social panics and repressive policies, is key for understanding today's hysterectomies.

In 1899, Dr. Magnus Hirschfeld, a medical doctor and sexologist in Berlin, published the first issue of *Jahrbuch für sexuelle Zwischenstufen* (*Yearbook for Intermediate Sexual Types*), an annual publication on same-sex desire and gender diversity that ran for twenty-five years. The *Jahrbuch* is where Hirschfeld first introduced his term *sexual intermediaries*, which refers to the idea that every person possesses "infinitely variable mixtures" of masculinity and femininity, arguing for a biological basis for gender and sexual variance.[56] In 1919, Hirschfeld founded the Institute for Sexual Science in Berlin, where he worked closely with the Austrian endocrinologist Eugene Steinach, the first to identify testosterone and estrogen and their associated effects on the body as "sex hormones." In collaboration, they began altering the bodies of patients who wished to transform their sex with surgeries and hormones.[57]

The momentum for Hirschfeld's work and hence the trans healthcare movement was halted by World War II. Hitler labeled Hirschfeld, who was gay, Jewish, and a vocal supporter of gay and trans rights, "the most dangerous Jew in Germany."[58] In 1933, the institute was raided and torched, and Hirschfeld was forced into exile in France, where he died in 1935. In her book, Stryker calls Hirschfeld "the linchpin, and his institute the hub, of the international network of transgender people and progressive medical experts who set the stage for the post–World War II transgender movement."[59]

Traction in trans health in the twentieth century was much slower in the United States relative to Europe. One early account is the story of Dr. Alan L. Hart, a medical doctor, who was the recipient of a hysterectomy by Dr. Joshua Allen Gilbert in 1917 in Oregon, as part of what's now understood as the first documented gender-affirming surgery in the United States.[60] In his 1920 journal article "Homo-Sexuality and Its Treatment," Gilbert cites painful menstruation and the "the inconvenience of dealing with this flow in male attire" as well as sterilization as the medical indications for this hysterectomy.[61] Gilbert also notes needing to be persuaded by Hart to perform the hysterectomy despite his "long hesitance and deliberation," but he came to see sterilization by hysterectomy as a sensible treatment to "her abnormal inversion."[62] A few decades later, in the 1940s and 1950s, some US-based research was conducted on sex and gender variance. However, the bulk of this research consisted of unethical experimentation using sex hormones and castration surgeries on imprisoned men in California penitentiaries and on outed gay men serving in the US Army.[63] These two early accounts of trans medicine in the United States showcase the influence of the eugenics movement as well as the pathologizing of sexual and gender "deviance" in the creation of trans medicine as we know it today.

Desired gender-affirming procedures in the United States, including hysterectomy, remained largely inaccessible, particularly because of widespread "mayhem" statutes across the country. Charges of mayhem could be leveled against any medical provider "unlawfully depriving a human being of a member of his or her body or disfiguring or rendering it useless," as defined in California's penal code.[64] It was not uncommon for some of these laws to include castration as a form of mayhem, such as in Texas: "Whoever willfully and maliciously deprives another person of either or both . . . of the testicles shall be confined in the penitentiary."[65] Whether or not mayhem laws applied to "sex reassignment surgeries," as they were called at the time, was a great source of legal debate even as late as the 1970s, though the fear of mayhem allegations created a chilling effect for many decades.[66] This historical legal framing of trans health as an unneeded disfigurement of the body helps contextualize today's hysterectomy stories, as many individuals have to prove their need for a hysterectomy in a medical system that continues to center cis patients while emphasizing fertility promotion of people with uteruses.

German-born Dr. Harry Benjamin, who worked closely with Hirschfeld and Steinach, was pivotal in finally developing trans healthcare in the United States, decades after European medicine had advanced the field. His book *The Transexual Phenomenon* (1966) not only popularized the term *transexual*—to distinguish it from *transvestite*—but also argued against doctors' attempts to "cure" transsexuals through psychotherapy.[67] At that time, it was a widespread belief in the United States that being trans constituted having a mental illness. For instance, the Supreme Court of New York case *Anonymous v. Weiner* (1966) ruled against granting a postoperative trans man a new birth certificate on the grounds that it would be "a means to help psychologically ill persons in their social adaptation."[68] Benjamin staunchly opposed the framing of transness as mental illness, and he soon became internationally known as the go-to surgeon for people seeking trans surgeries. In 1979, he created the International Gender Dysphoria Association, which published yearly standards of care in trans health. The association was renamed in 2009 as the World Professional Association for Transgender Health, and its ongoing publication of standards of care remains critical to the field of trans health and continues to define the provision of hysterectomy for trans and nonbinary patients.

The hysterectomy stories in this book reflect this historical tension between trans healthcare and the fields of psychology and psychiatry. I write this chapter only fifteen years after the 2009 call for the depathologization and depsychologization of gender variance among a variety of entities in Europe and the United States. It was not until 2013 that the *Diagnostic and Statistical Manual of Mental Disorders* (*DSM*) finally changed its classification from "sexual and gender identity disorders" to "gender dysphoria," which, while still contentious, moves the clinical focus away from transness itself to the feeling of discomfort experienced by trans people. Medical gatekeeping of gender-affirming care is also an enduring issue, with providers wielding the power to determine who is "truly" trans or in need of surgery and hormone therapy, which, as in the twentieth century, has the greatest impact on trans people who were assigned female at birth.[69]

Despite the lack of a similar scientific momentum toward trans healthcare in the United States compared with Europe, there was nonetheless demonstrated desire for this care. In 1953, Christine Jorgensen—a US citizen and World War II veteran—underwent genital reconstruction surgery in Denmark. Jorgensen's surgery sparked international headlines, and she quickly became a media sensation, which then introduced the notion of sex mutability to the United States.[70] With new language to describe a pervasive feeling of discomfort with one's sex and assigned gender, a wave of Americans seeking gender-affirming care in Denmark ensued, eventually leading to a ban on such procedures for non-Danish citizens. Today's hysterectomy stories continue to reflect a geography-based access to trans care, which requires many trans and nonbinary people to engage in medical tourism across state (or national) lines to access needed procedures like hysterectomy.

When the first gender identity clinic to offer gender-affirming surgery in the United States opened at Johns Hopkins University Hospital in 1965, it received upwards of two thousand requests for care. In the fourteen years the clinic was open, only twenty-four patients were treated, given the clinic's strong preference for candidates who were most likely to "pass" as the opposite sex and adhere to normative gendered expectations. The clinic shut down amid anti-trans controversy.[71] Hysterectomy patients today are often expected to adhere to a standard of care trajectory, which in many cases begins with a gender dysphoria evaluation by a mental health provider. Within these evaluations, as in the Johns Hopkins clinic of the 1960s, there is an emphasis on binary trans identities and adherence to normative gender roles, in a way that excludes gender-nonconforming and nonbinary experiences. Over fifty years later, many of the issues that led the first trans health clinic to shut down continue to haunt today's trans healthcare, as reflected in contemporary hysterectomy stories.

It should be noted that gender-affirming procedures like hysterectomy were neither novel nor unique to trans people. On the contrary, these were common procedures long performed on cis men and women, yet they were deemed controversial when requested or performed for gendered reasons. Dr. Nikolaj Bogoraz, a Russian surgeon, performed the first known total phalloplasty (the surgical construction of a penis) on a twenty-three-year-old cis man who had suffered a traumatic injury (to be more precise, his wife cut off his penis while he was asleep).[72] Phalloplasty was then widely used as a reconstructive procedure for soldiers wounded in World War I. Oophorectomy (removal of one or both ovaries) and mastectomy were similarly not new procedures but, rather, part of the development of early surgery. There are records of mastectomy being used for breast tumors as early as the sixteenth century. In 1895, the Scottish surgeon George Beatson discovered that oophorectomy shrank breast tumors, leading to a widespread practice of ovary excision to treat breast cancer.[73] Hormone replacement therapy was also long used to treat cis men and women for a wide range of endocrine issues, from hypogonadism to menopause.[74]

Historical and contemporary hesitancy, then—or outright refusal—to perform these same treatments on trans people is often not rooted in lack of technical knowledge or surgical skill. Hysterectomy is merely one of many procedures that began as part of medical care for cisgender people but came to take on new social meanings, stigmas, and moral panics when integrated into trans health.

The wave of anti-trans bills currently coursing through the country's state and county legislatures seek to return to a fully pathologized model of transness, in contradiction of decades of scientific research. These bills aim to reframe gender-affirming care as harmful, and trans patients as victims of the medical-industrial complex, neglectful parenting, and/or exploitative social media trends. However, regressive forces have long tried to suppress trans communities, but even the Nazi regime burning down Hirschfeld's institute couldn't stop the progression of trans healthcare. As the stories in this book will show, the field of trans medicine continues to move forward, showcasing incredible resilience as trans patients reshape medicine from within.

LOOKING FORWARD: WEAVING TOGETHER THESE HISTORIES

While these histories—the emergence of gynecology, medical abuse conducted and enabled selectively by race, and the development of trans healthcare—tend to be thought of as existing on separate planes, they are inextricably linked. Without the professionalization of medicine and surgical methods spearheaded by gynecology, there would be no trans healthcare; more disturbingly, without the exploitation and abuse of Black and brown people in the United States and abroad, it's difficult to imagine where the field of gynecology would be today. By examining these different stories and seeing the parallel ways history unfolded by gender and race, we can better understand contemporary patterns—regarding hysterectomy but also expanding far beyond this procedure.

Hysterectomy is the missing piece linking together these dark histories in medicine. Analyzing contemporary understandings and uses of the hysterectomy yields critical insight into the mechanizations of modern medicine, gender stratification, and racism in medicine. In the abstract and when stripped of social context, hysterectomy is not inherently good or bad, morally or otherwise, but nevertheless has been used as a symbolic receptacle for a wide range of cultural meanings and values.

The next chapters invite the reader to consider the following questions: How do modern hysterectomy stories reflect these interlinked histories? How does a person's identity shape their experience in the clinic and in the operating room? And more broadly, what can we learn about medicine, gender, and reproduction from hysterectomy—a surgery whose provision is shaped by years of racism and adherence to the gender binary?

HISTORICAL TIMELINE

50 BC First recorded vaginal hysterectomy, performed by Themison of Athens

120 Vaginal hysterectomy on an inverted uterus, performed by Soranus of Ephesus

1809 First surgical opening of abdomen

1843 First abdominal hysterectomy, performed by Charles Clay in Manchester, England. Misdiagnosis led to the patient's immediate death postoperatively

1845–49 Dr. J. Marion Sims performs surgical experiments on enslaved women in Montgomery, Alabama (including Anarcha, Betsey, and Lucy); develops the duckbill (aka "Sims") speculum

1853 First nonfatal abdominal hysterectomy, performed by Ellis Burnham of Lowell, Massachusetts

1853 First "deliberate hysterectomy" using anesthesia for a fibroid, performed by Gilman Kimball of Massachusetts

1863 First successful hysterectomy with oophorectomy and salpingectomy, performed by Charles Clay

1899 Dr. Magnus Hirschfeld publishes the first issue of *Yearbook for Intermediate Sexual Types*

1908 Endometriosis first identified by the Canadian gynecologist Thomas Cullen

1909 California passes its first law on nonconsensual sterilizations, beginning its seventy-year eugenics movement

1912 Early account of hysterectomy for a female-to-male trans person in Berlin

1919 Dr. Magnus Hirschfeld founds the Institute for Sexual Science in Berlin

1917 Alan L. Hart receives a hysterectomy as part of the first documented gender-affirming surgery in the United States

1920s Transverse incision introduced by Johanns Pfannenstiel, making hysterectomies safer

1921 Dr. John Sampson, an American gynecologist, proposes the cause of "retrograde menstruation," naming it "endometriosis"

1927 *Buck v. Bell* affirms state-enforced sterilization to "prevent those who are manifestly unfit from continuing their kind"

1929 The first total abdominal hysterectomy to avoid the risk of cervical carcinoma developing is performed by E. H. Richardson in the United States

1930 The governor of Puerto Rico, Menendez Ramos, implements forced sterilization programs for Puerto Rican women

1932 The USPHS Untreated Syphilis Study at Tuskegee (previously called the Tuskegee Study of Untreated Syphilis in the Negro Male) and widely known as the Tuskegee Experiment, begins at the Tuskegee Institute in Macon, Alabama

1933 The Nazi regime burns down the Institute for Sexual Science

1949 Harry Benjamin begins to treat transgender individuals in San Francisco with hormones

1951 Doctors take Henrietta Lacks's cervical tissue for research without her consent

1952 Christine Jorgensen undergoes sex reassignment surgery in Copenhagen and returns to unauthorized media reports of her story in the United States

1952 The American Psychiatric Association officially drops the term *hysteria* along with 250 "hystero-neurasthenic disorders" from the canon of modern disease paradigms

1960–70 Sterilization abuse of Black women in the United States reaches record levels

1964 Reed Erickson, a wealthy trans man, founds the Erickson Educational Foundation, which funded research on "transsexuality"

1966 Johns Hopkins University Hospital, with funds from Erickson, announces its gender identity clinic to provide sex reassignment surgery

1969 Stonewall Riots begin the gay rights movement

1970–76 25–50 percent of Native Americans are forcibly sterilized

1970 *Roe v. Wade* codifies the constitutional right to an abortion

1972 Tuskegee Experiment is ended

1974 US Supreme Court hears *Relf v. Weinberger*; finds coercive sterilization unconstitutional

1975 Class action lawsuit is brought against Southern California Hospitals for nonconsensual sterilization procedures on residents of the predominantly Latine Los Angeles district

1976 Tennis ace Reneé Richards is outed and barred from competition when she attempts to enter a women's tennis tournament. Her subsequent legal battle establishes that in the United States, trans individuals are legally accepted in their new identity after reassignment

1979 California repeals its involuntary sterilization law following more than twenty thousand sterilizations

1988 First laparoscopic hysterectomy performed by Harry Reich in Kingston, Pennsylvania

1993 "Don't Ask Don't Tell" policy is instituted for gay, lesbian, and bisexual service members

1998 Hystersisters.com started, still one of the most prominent sources of information and support for hysterectomy patients

2004 The Gender Recognition Act becomes law, allowing transgender persons to legally change their sex and have it recognized for marriage and other purposes

2011 "Don't Ask Don't Tell" policy is repealed

2016 Pentagon lifts the ban on transgender people serving openly in the US armed services

2016 "Bathroom bill controversy" in North Carolina begins conversations about using public restrooms associated with one's gender identity

2017 Trump administration issues a formal memorandum to ban transgender people from the US armed services

2018 Lena Dunham writes about her wanted hysterectomy at age thirty-one for *Vogue* magazine

2020 Allegations are publicized of forced hysterectomies for detained women in ICE camps

2021 Record number of anti-trans bills introduced in the US South

2021 Texas's Senate Bill 8, or SB8, the most extreme antiabortion bill in recent US history, passes into law

2022 Governor Greg Abbott of Texas calls for investigations into parents of trans children who have received gender-affirming care

2022 US Supreme Court overturns *Roe v. Wade*

2

WHY WOULD SOMEONE WANT A HYSTERECTOMY?

How do I feel about my uterus? It'd been torturing me for years.

Thus began my interview with Lee, a twenty-nine-year-old white nonbinary artist living in Arizona. Freshly two weeks after their hysterectomy, Lee shared their story with me over Zoom, settled into a couch in the living room they share with their partner. Since their first menstrual period at age thirteen, Lee has dealt with endometriosis in addition to the chronic illness fibromyalgia, which some studies have found tends to co-occur with endometriosis for reasons that remain mysterious.[1] While hormonal birth control masked Lee's endometriosis symptoms throughout most of their adolescence, they began to feel something was "wrong" by age eighteen and told their gynecologist, "I have pelvic pain. It doesn't feel quite right down there." After that, Lee's symptoms went into turbo mode, and every three months they would have a menstrual period so painful they were throwing up in the bathroom and calling in sick to work. By the time they turned twenty-three, Lee told me, "Every time I ovulated and every time I had a period, I was so sick."

Lee's symptoms were ignored and undiagnosed for thirteen years; the gynecologist Lee saw for eleven years told them repeatedly, "Oh it's just a period, honey." Their path to healing began not with their doctor but during a conversation with a friend when they were twenty-six. This was the first time Lee heard the word *endometriosis* and began to consider whether this condition might be the source of their problems. Lee's friend strongly recommended an endometriosis specialist; despite endometriosis impacting roughly 10 percent of people with uteruses, gynecology regards this condition, along with other illnesses that affect the uterus and ovaries, as necessitating specialized knowledge and training. Since surgery is currently the only way to diagnose endometriosis (although it was discovered in 1860 and named in 1925),[2] Lee's journey then led them to the operating room. "I came out of anesthesia and immediately asked for my partner and my mom. And my first question was, 'Did they find it?'" After over a decade of dealing with an unnamed, mysterious illness that was upending their life, Lee decided they'd had enough, and a hysterectomy to remove the source of their pain was next. The way they describe wanting this surgery is emblematic of how many of the hysterectomy seekers I spoke to talk about their hysterectomy:

> I didn't go into it thinking, like, "Oh, I'll have a hysterectomy and I'll be cured." Like, I have a chronic illness and like, I'm still trying to figure out my body right now. But just the idea that I could have a hysterectomy felt like a tool in my toolbox. And to not utilize it would be detrimental to myself. And if you have a tool, why not use it?

Lee discusses a hysterectomy as something that one opts into as a way to care for oneself—a tool in the toolbox. The decision to have an "elective" hysterectomy like Lee's problematizes the binary that is typically applied to health procedures as either *lifesaving* or *elective*. In choosing to have one's uterus removed, most people, like Lee, aren't choosing between life or death, but rather between a life in pain or a life worth living. Such a choice reflects a cultural shift toward the biomedicalization of everything about us—of using the biomedical tools at our disposal to improve our lives in some way, rather than simply to save our lives.[3] When you begin looking for it, biomedicalization is everywhere: in Botox injections and hair transplants, in cochlear implants and hearing aids, in prosthetic limbs and titanium hips. Hysterectomy patients like Lee are therefore making this choice in a biomedicalized world where "health" is a commodity, and a body transformed by technoscience is a "prized possession."[4] A hysterectomy is sought to enhance or "fix" the body, forge or affirm an identity, mitigate symptoms or risk of illness—or all of the above. To not seek such a tool in this context, as Lee says, would be detrimental.

The usefulness of hysterectomy, however, was discussed differently depending on whether the person sought a hysterectomy to manage chronic illness or as part of trans medicine (there were only sixteen of the forty-six interviewees who fit into both groups). For those whose uterus caused significant illness, hysterectomy is a solution to a defective uterus or broken body; for those seeking a hysterectomy for trans health, it's a solution to a pesky or extraneous organ, or an inconvenient organ that should not have been there in the first place. These ways of thinking about the uterus and its removal shed light not only on how biomedicalization functions but also on how historically misused "tools" like hysterectomy are reclaimed by patients the medical system has long neglected.

"MY UTERUS DOESN'T WORK"

The uterus has wreaked havoc on the lives of many of the people described in this book. In interviews, participants with chronic illness described extreme symptoms that significantly interfered with their lives: from pain so severe, they had to lie down on the floor in the middle of the workday, to bleeding so heavy they needed multiple layers of pads, tampons, and sometimes adult diapers. These symptoms hindered their ability to work, travel, attend school, parent, date and have relationships, and have a social life. It is curious, then, that the one sociological book on hysterectomy details stories of grief about *losing* menstruation.[5] Surely, for some, to have a period is a source of pride or strength. But the romanticization of menstruation—or even of pregnancy and birth—will never reflect everyone's experience, particularly those for whom menstruation brings pain or gender dysphoria. Instead, for people for whom this organ brings disturbance or suffering, the uterus and its various functions often conjure the phrase "I just want it out."

Across interviews with people with chronic illness, many went beyond describing their pain and suffering as a form of sickness to evoking language of brokenness or defectiveness in their bodies and particularly of their uteruses. They used a range of metaphors to describe this brokenness—a broken machine part, a Swiss cheese organ, even a car window that no longer rolls down and is not in use. These self-assessments often came after years of their symptoms being normalized by doctors, family members, and ultimately themselves. Consider Tyesha, a fifty-year-old Black woman who grew up in Central Texas and is living in Alabama, where she attends graduate school and works as a research assistant at a hospital. From her first period at the age of thirteen, she had adenomyosis symptoms that she and her parents attributed to part of normal menstruation. "I thought everyone had horrible periods," she told me. "They were painful, they were heavy. I didn't know much about period variation, I just knew that they were awful for me." She said that growing up, she would have to run to the bathroom during class to change her tampons and pads every hour or two, and as an adult had to miss days at work due to the pain—"because I literally could not get out of bed." Tyesha was finally diagnosed with adenomyosis and fibroids at the age of thirty-three after experiencing a miscarriage. After that, she had various treatments and surgeries to try to get her symptoms under control, including years taking hormonal birth control, the removal of her left ovary, a myomectomy for fibroid removal, and a hematoma evacuation as a result of a complication from the myomectomy.

In describing her uterus and ovaries, Tyesha said, "My internal organs felt like a chemistry set and it's like, we're trying to work, but we can't work." After continuing to experience immense pain and bleeding even after multiple treatments and surgeries, she started to think about a hysterectomy and talked to her ob-gyn "about let's get it out." When I asked what she was thinking as she first began to consider the hysterectomy, she said, "It was too much. It was too much pain and too many accidents. . . . I was weighing whether or not I wanted to bleed all the time and be in this much pain versus just get it out." She ended up having a hysterectomy, including the removal of her right ovary, and she said that afterward she felt "lighter" and like she had one fewer thing she had to "mentally triage."

Margot's path, like that of thousands of other women in the United States, was similar to Tyesha's. A forty-one-year-old white woman living with her husband in Virginia, where she works in media strategy and sales, Margot has experienced extreme bouts of pain and excessive bleeding since her first menstrual period at the age of fifteen. These "episodes" could happen at any moment, severely disrupting her life. She recounted a particularly distressing occurrence in public, where her usual coping strategies led to suspicion rather than concern from those around her followed by her own deep embarrassment:

> I had an episode in Ikea. I felt it coming on and I was like, "Uh-oh, here it comes." I just had to go sit in the Ikea bathroom, just rocking back and forth. I found the formula when I was a teenager, if I just hmm, the vibrations would make things calm down and it would exhaust me. But doing that in a public place with a bunch of strangers looking at me like they thought I was a drug addict or something, it's such an emotional and mental struggle because you want to be able to say, "No, I'm just sick with this period," but you can't verbalize it.

Margot spent her teenage years in and out of doctors' offices seeking relief from symptoms of what was later diagnosed as adenomyosis. The solutions presented were always a different form of hormonal birth control, which lessened the bleeding but not the pain. Prior to this diagnosis, doctors repeatedly told her what she was experiencing was normal; they suggested she was "very sensitive," which led Margot to believe "maybe I'm just dramatic." When she was in her thirties, she sought an IUD to manage her symptoms, but her doctor had difficulty placing the device due to the irregular shape of her uterus. Margot told me about how she felt that day at the doctor's office, after the extremely painful—and unsuccessful—attempt at relief via an IUD:

I started crying, and I was just like, I'm broken. I am broken. I am a broken person. My uterus doesn't work. I have all these problems. It's so frustrating. I don't want to be just looked at as a reproductive machine, but at the same time my reproductive system doesn't work and it's an issue.

Like Margot, participants with chronic illness often felt that along with being "broken," they were simultaneously struggling against the normative idea of motherhood as destiny—or, as Margot put it, of women being "reproductive machines." At the time of our interview, Margot had not had a hysterectomy, but she thought about it frequently; she had put it off for years in the hope that "research would catch up," but new biomedical advancements never materialized. Now, at forty-one, fed up with her symptoms and with no desire to try for a pregnancy, she said the time for her hysterectomy might finally have arrived.

Evoking a variation on the metaphor of brokenness, incompleteness, or distortedness, Yerma described their uterus as "a Swiss cheese uterus." Yerma is a thirty-seven-year-old, white, agender elementary school teacher living in New York, who until recently identified as a heterosexual cisgender woman. They described having severe menstrual symptoms that started at the age of nineteen and became more debilitating over time. "My body's all fucked up," is how Yerma began recounting their history with endometriosis. Throughout their life, Yerma experienced pelvic pain, heavy bleeding, anemia, painful sex, and repeated miscarriages. At the peak of their symptoms in their early thirties, Yerma was so anemic they were passing out in public, including one time they woke up at a bus station in Brooklyn in the middle of winter. Life was "starting to get really dark," they told me. Yerma had always wanted to gestate a pregnancy and have a large family with their husband, but they ultimately felt this would be impossible and became increasingly interested in a hysterectomy, which they finally had at the age of thirty-six—seventeen years after their symptoms began—after pleading with various doctors. They told me, "I had a fucked-up like totally like Swiss cheese uterus. It had to go. It was not a working organ. It was a broken organ, but it's amazing how people don't want you to take it out." Despite their doctors insisting that nothing was wrong with them and that a pregnancy would be possible, Yerma firmly believed their uterus was "a broken organ." As it turns out, their instinct was right. After going to a specialist and undergoing exploratory surgery, they were diagnosed with highly progressed endometriosis and adenomyosis, both of which had warped their uterus and rendered a pregnancy highly improbable.

For some, a desire for a hysterectomy is accompanied by a desire to not have children, rendering the elective sterilization aspect of the procedure a benefit. One such woman is Hallie, a twenty-five-year-old white woman working as a child psychologist in rural South Carolina, where she lives with her husband. She has endometriosis, with periods that sometimes last up to twenty-one days. Given her illness and the decision she and her husband have made to live a "child-free life," she described her uterus as a broken part within her body akin to a car's broken window. She tried various forms of birth control but ultimately decided that none sufficiently managed her symptoms, after which she repeatedly told her doctor, "Just take it out." Describing her journey leading to a hysterectomy at twenty-four, and how she felt about her uterus, she said:

> We discovered that I also had endometriosis and some other problems. My uterus was misshapen and other things. So, we tried hormonal treatments for about a year, a year-and-a-half. And then nothing really made it . . . I mean, stuff made it *better*, but nothing ever made it to a place of like, "Yes, I can spend the rest of my life at this level." It's like having a broken window in your car. The back passenger window doesn't go down anymore. You never use that window. And you don't have any plans to use that window.

As this quote highlights, people like Hallie often described their bodies or their uteruses as broken, and a hysterectomy as a solution to make their lives more *livable*. Stories like this underscore how the tools of medicine, like hysterectomy, can be transformed not only by technical advancements but also by evolving meanings attached to "health" and to bodies. At the end of our interview Hallie said, "It's not the end of the world. . . . Yes, it is a major surgery. But you have to do what you have to do to be happy and to be healthy."

Many also viewed a hysterectomy as a way to be better people for those around them—a biomedicalized solution in order to engage more fully in social roles. For instance, Anjali is a twenty-eight-year-old South Asian woman who lives in California, where she works as a therapist and is raising her young daughter with her husband. She told me that she sought a hysterectomy in order to be a better partner, mother, and employee. She described how she came to have a hysterectomy after years of debilitating endometriosis symptoms that were drastically interfering with her life. Growing up, the pain she experienced caused fainting and trips to the emergency room, and she missed so much school she had to attend summer school to catch up. And yet, it took ten years to begin to get "proper care." "My parents are just very . . . in Indian culture, it's still very stigmatized, periods," she told me. "The whole talk around it. It was never really talked about until my pain got so bad, and it became more evident and that it stemmed from my uterus."

After a decade of pain, Anjali decided to have a hysterectomy. She said, "I never really desired one, but then at a point, when it was told to me that this was the only cure, I was like, 'I'm ready,' because my life was so . . . I wasn't able to function as a person." Notably, though the surgery was a choice for Anjali, it was not an entirely free choice—rather, it is a constrained choice. As she and others discuss, hysterectomy is often the *only* option for relief amid a medical system that has neglected to invest in understanding the diseases of the uterus.

Shaping the desire toward the constrained choice of a hysterectomy is surgery's modern transformation into a procedure that entails a few small incisions and often does not even require an overnight stay at the hospital. This shift from invasive to "minimally invasive" was key in Maty's decision to pursue her surgery. Maty is a fifty-three-year-old Hispanic woman living in California, where she raised three children with her husband and works as a commercial property manager. Maty had fibroids for years; at the age of forty-two she learned that hysterectomy, the only permanent solution to fibroids, could be an outpatient procedure performed without extensive cutting or suturing. The following is her description of how she learned of the hysterectomy as a solution, as well as her thought process regarding why a hysterectomy is an ideal—albeit constrained—choice for other people with chronic issues like her own:

> I was like, "Okay, so you don't have to cut me open?" And [the surgeon] said, "I don't think so unless there's a complication." So, we set it up. And it was really easy. I don't know why more people don't do it. I really don't. I personally don't understand if [the uterus] causes so many problems in women, why would we keep something that we are no longer going to use? . . . I don't understand why we have to keep it. I really don't.

Maty's words capture the joint construction of the modern hysterectomy: it no longer is the invasive, dangerous procedure it always was, and people are also increasingly understanding the uterus as something they do not have a self-evident use for. Instead, in our modern biomedicalized era, if a uterus is causing problems, removing it can come to be viewed as the necessary option, a prudent decision—and, in many cases, the only choice.

THE BIG SCOOP: HYSTERECTOMY AS SELF-CARE

Trans and nonbinary hysterectomy seekers likewise view this surgery as a tool for "taking care of themselves." Hysterectomy is often understood within the transmasculine community—by providers and patients alike—as a preventive measure and a way of staying "healthy."[6] Rather than to alleviate current physical symptoms, however, a hysterectomy is often sought out to prevent the possibility of future illness that could be caused by long-term exposure to testosterone. Accordingly, many of the trans and nonbinary people I interviewed described the uterus more along the lines of an annoying or extraneous organ that was not meant to be there in the first place. Many even forget or ignore the uterus altogether unless they are actively bleeding or cramping (testosterone typically eliminates menstruation). And yet, others wanted a hysterectomy to permanently remove the possibility of menstruation, "breakthrough" occurrences of bleeding or cramping, pregnancy, and the need for gynecological exams—all of which can induce gender dysphoria. A hysterectomy as part of trans health, then, touches on all the cornerstones of biomedicalization, in that it is used to achieve a sense of "health and wellness," to forge or affirm a new embodied identity, as well as to prevent risk of future disease.

For those following the WPATH standards of care manual, the guide says under "Risks of Masculinizing Hormone Therapy" that ovarian and endometrial cancer present "inconclusive or no increased risk," and that they "may present risk, but for which the evidence is so minimal that no clear conclusion can be reached."[7] This evidence is based on small case studies rather than well-designed, longitudinal epidemiological studies. Yet those who are prone to health anxiety might read into this ambiguity and conclude they should have a hysterectomy as a form of self-care—especially if a doctor is recommending it. Jax, for instance, is a thirty-two-year-old white trans man living in a large city in Illinois, where he works as a social worker. He began his journey with gender-affirming healthcare when he was twenty, and his first priorities were top surgery and testosterone. Twelve years later, he hasn't had a hysterectomy, because menstruation ended with testosterone use and he doesn't think about his uterus much. However, Jax continues to weigh having the procedure, as he, along with many others, understand it as a tool to achieve health and well-being. He told me:

> I did not and have not had a lot of dysphoria around my uterus, but I definitely want to be on top of my health. That's important to me. And so, I wondered is this something that I need to do? And for a while the message that I got was, "Yes, this is something that you should do. We don't really know for sure. But why not, you know, be on the safe side or whatever?" So that was when I started thinking more about it.

Rather than being a tool to alleviate gender dysphoria, then, a hysterectomy has been on Jax's to-do list for years as a form of preventative health and to "be on top of" his health.

Similarly, Hal, a thirty-six-year-old white trans man living in Alaska, where he co-parents a foster son with his wife, explained his thought process for wanting a hysterectomy:

> I didn't think about hysterectomy too much until I started testosterone. And my doctor had said, "Hey, there's not a lot of studies on what long-term testosterone use does to female reproductive organs—eventually you're going to want to get those taken out." So I was like, OK, well, I'll get that eventually, top surgery is what I really want now, having a large chest and not wanting to be someone with a chest, with boobs, that was what I really wanted first. So, yeah, we prioritized that within the first year.

As Hal and many others explained, the desire for a hysterectomy was often spurred by being told it is an important health step for those taking testosterone for the long term, despite the limited research and contradictory opinions. Meanwhile, other elements of trans health, like testosterone or top surgery, were prioritized over hysterectomy given the more visible benefits.

Stewart is another person who was long confused by the conflicting messages he and many other transmasculine individuals receive about a hysterectomy. He is a thirty-four-year-old white trans man living with his girlfriend in a midsize city in Colorado, where he works as a grocery store worker. Stewart ultimately chose a hysterectomy as a precautionary measure, after balancing multiple streams of medical advice:

> I wasn't sure about hysterectomy, except that I figured it was kind of a necessary progression, because not just for dysphoria reasons, but because of some people were saying and who knows, because there's no information. Some people were saying, "OK, as long as you have ovaries and stuff, it's conflicting with the testosterone." And then some people are saying, "[The uterus is] going to atrophy on testosterone eventually and it could become cancerous as it's not active tissue maybe, but it could take years." And then some people were saying, "It doesn't matter."

As these comments indicate, while a hysterectomy is regarded by the medical community as a "gender-affirming procedure," the extent to which a hysterectomy can or does affirm gender varies. Mac, a twenty-six-year-old white trans man who is a college student in New York, told me, "I needed top surgery to be taken seriously as a man, but no one knows whether I have a uterus or not." Similarly, Brian views a distinction between the benefits of hysterectomy and other elements of trans health. Brian is a twenty-three-year-old biracial Asian American trans man living in New Jersey, where he attends graduate school, who compared his reasons for wanting a hysterectomy versus top surgery as follows:

Top surgery is more of like a physical change to how people would see me and how I would see myself versus like me getting some internal organ out. I imagine one would be better for my body than the other. So like whereas hysterectomy would be like, good for me because I would be like, lessening my chance of cancer, a top surgery would just be like I want this to affirm my gender.

For Brian and others, then, a hysterectomy is desired for a healthy body, rather than solely or primarily for gender affirmation.

Still others desired a hysterectomy to feel more aligned with their gender identity. Gabri, a twenty-five-year-old Mexican American nonbinary person who grew up in rural North Carolina, never quite felt comfortable in their body. In their conservative Catholic family, Gabri was always considered rebellious—for not liking wearing dresses, not "sitting properly," and being too sporty. When they finally learned the words during college to describe their experiences and desires—words like *gender dysphoria*, *nonbinary*, and *transgender*—they decided to seek gender-affirming healthcare. The first priority on the list for Gabri was top surgery, and they started a GoFundMe page to crowdsource the money for the procedure. For Gabri and many others in this book, the external physicality of top surgery made it more of a priority over the benefits of a hysterectomy, which aren't visible; for example, top surgery grants a newfound freedom to take off one's shirt at the beach and to have a flat chest without having to wear an often-uncomfortable binder. Such embodied benefits of top surgery made Gabri want to continue on their journey with gender-affirming care—moving on to taking testosterone, and then beginning to consider a hysterectomy as their next step. When I asked what led them to first seriously consider a hysterectomy, they told me, "I'm going to get like everything done that I possibly can to make me feel more in tune with my body to feel more comfortable with myself."

The notion of seeking a hysterectomy to feel more in tune with one's body or more comfortable with one's identity is emblematic of a hysterectomy as a tool in the toolbox. While the definition of "health" for those with chronic illness is clear—removal of the main source of pain and bleeding—it becomes more complicated for those forging a new gender identity with the aid of technoscientific approaches. Health in this case is not only physical but also psychological and symbolic, and surgery emerges as a way to feel better. In a different part of the interview, Gabri mentioned that they had never had a gynecological visit, initially because of a lack of health insurance (their family is undocumented) and later because of a fear of being nonbinary in a feminized healthcare space.[8] By having a hysterectomy, Gabri told me, they hoped they would be able to avoid both the need for routine gynecological visits, which include pap smears, as well as the risk of forgoing such visits. Stories like Gabri's showcase how access to gender-affirming care like hysterectomy is strongly associated with a range of improved physical and mental health outcomes. With one surgery, Gabri feels affirmed in their gender, can avoid the anxiety of gynecological exams, and averts potential risk of illness that could arise from avoiding medical care.

Appreciating the immense benefits gender-affirming care can bring, many of my interviewees shared Gabri's desire to do everything possible to inch closer toward this notion of health and wellness. In this light, the prospect of getting a hysterectomy has some appeal given the various mental health benefits of gender-affirming care. Like Gabri, Jax, mentioned earlier, described wanting to get everything done that he possibly can to maximize these mental health benefits: "I first thought about a hysterectomy after starting T[estosterone], and I was like, I wonder if this is possible. I was looking up all the surgeries . . . like all the surgery, I was like, well, what can I do here?" As prior medical sociologists, including stef shuster and Georgiann Davis, have demonstrated, the process of accessing trans medicine often involves a series of bureaucratic hurdles and structural obstacles.[9] After years of grappling with one's potential trans identity, one then has to navigate a complicated healthcare system: finding providers who are knowledgeable and affirming, (often) getting a gender dysphoria diagnosis, and fulfilling various therapeutic and psychological requirements, not to mention finding the financial means and/or insurance coverage necessary for any of the aforementioned. After these navigations, many patients are eager to obtain as many procedures as possible, or to at least feel as if they are optimizing all available choices.

For some, the prospect of a hysterectomy was highly gender-affirming in and of itself, as it removes bodily and social processes generally associated with femininity and womanhood. Some experienced gender dysphoria from menstruating, and others from the mere thought of pregnancy (though, of course, this is not the case for all trans and nonbinary people). Hysterectomy in these cases can therefore be a tool to remove the biological and social roles of the uterus. For instance, Jeff, a twenty-three-year-old queer white trans man from Virginia now living in California, remembers feeling uncomfortable when he first learned about the uterus during sex education. He told me, "I tried really hard not to think about the fact that I personally had a uterus because the idea of getting pregnant made me really uncomfortable." While he sought a hysterectomy primarily to manage endometriosis symptoms, he also welcomed the removal of the possibility of pregnancy, for gender-affirming reasons. Likewise, Enrique, a twenty-two-year-old mixed-race (white, Latino) trans man in New York, says his primary motivation for a hysterectomy is his doctor's recommendation as a health precaution. However, it would also be gender-affirming, since he has never wanted to become pregnant. He told me:

Even before realizing I was trans, I knew from a really young age I never wanted to give birth. I was quite uncomfortable with my uterus's existence, and the association with having a uterus means you have to be a woman and all of that. I was not having it.

Echoing this, Semyon, a twenty-nine-year-old white gay trans man in New York, told me, "The idea of being pregnant was always extremely dysphoria inducing and unpleasant to me." As someone who has sex with cis men, no longer having to worry about pregnancy prevention after the hysterectomy was gender-affirming.

Aiden is a twenty-nine-year-old white agender person living in a city in California who had a hysterectomy at twenty-eight as part of seeking gender-affirming healthcare. Aiden is one of a handful of interviewees who, like Semyon, sought a hysterectomy exclusively for gender-affirming reasons; they did not discuss a desire to reduce cancer risk or problems with breakthrough bleeding and cramping from taking testosterone. Like many trans and nonbinary people, Aiden dreaded the physical experiences that a uterus can confer—particularly menstruation and pregnancy. But beyond that anxiety, Aiden was "horrified" by the fact of having a uterus. They told me, "As soon as I found out, probably in the fifth grade, that I had a uterus and what it was for, I pretty much immediately went, 'No, do not want.' I was horrified and really not okay with that." As they told me:

> I didn't want my uterus, that organ inside of me. Well, it had everything to do with reproduction. The whole menstruation thing is just a pain in the ass. I think nobody likes it, it's a bad idea, it's inconvenient, it's messy, it's another logistics to deal with. But I really didn't want to be able to reproduce. I was in terror of that happening, of getting pregnant, being unable to get an abortion, having to carry to term. That all got worse with the 2016 election. It was a pervasive anxiety and, yeah, just the thought of it horrified me.

Hysterectomy is therefore not only a way to minimize the risk of cancer (which can kill you) but also to minimize the risk of pregnancy (which, statistically, can also kill you, in addition to causing gender dysphoria and now being difficult to terminate post-*Dobbs*). This case therefore deepens our understanding of biomedicalization by showing that biomedicine not only can be gendered but also can be used to evade previous gendered expectations and forge new gender categories altogether.

Mac, who calls his hysterectomy "the big scoop," explained to me the various ways it was beneficial to his life and overall health:

> I didn't want to get pregnant. I didn't want to have things in there that I just really didn't want to have . . . this extra organ I really didn't need. I felt it was more symbolic of something that I wasn't. You know, like, you can have a uterus and be a man. Like, that's no problem. But I was like, *I* want it gone. Especially because it was causing so much pain. I'm very grateful that I had it [removed]. I don't have to worry about cramping anymore. All the pain is gone. So I feel great. I never wanted it in the first place. And I call the hysto the big scoop. And the big scoop solved all that for me.

Mac and others acknowledge that they believe body parts and gender can and should be uncoupled—"you can have a uterus and be a man"—yet many still felt a desire to customize their own body via the removal of this organ. In these cases, the "health" status associated with the hysterectomy was typically in terms of mental health and the psychological relief that comes with feeling affirmed with one's gender. Mac's comments also encapsulate a key difference in how people with chronic illness and transmasculine people talk about their uterus—for the former, the uterus is broken or defective, and for the latter, the uterus was extraneous, erroneous, and "never wanted." In both cases, however, the hysterectomy, or big scoop, is a tool in the toolbox to achieve biomedicalized health goals. Beyond strictly treating current or possible illness, a hysterectomy can also be *chosen* as a tool to achieve a new definition of health: a state of feeling in harmony with yourself.

FINDING RELIEF IN A SYSTEM BUILT FOR HAVING BABIES

People who come to want a hysterectomy as a technofix are desiring this surgery amid broader cultural and systemic failures. Whether to treat chronic illness or as part of trans healthcare, patients are choosing hysterectomy in a culture that normalizes pain as part of having a uterus, and one that centers cisgender identities. Not to mention, a hysterectomy is chosen within a medical system that is oriented around cis women who want to birth babies and thus neglects other health concerns of the uterus and ovaries. The very sector that deals with "women's health" within the National Institutes of Health (NIH), for instance, is called the National Institute of Child Health and Human Development (NICHD), which effectively erases the people who get pregnant and have children. Of the paltry 10 percent of the NIH research budget that goes to "women's health," a full 80 percent is dedicated to pregnancy and childbirth research—meaning only 2 percent of the budget goes toward researching health issues like endometriosis, fibroids, and uterine prolapse. The experiences of hysterectomy seekers reflect medicine's hyperfocus on fertility and the dangers of neglecting the other functions and needs of a body that houses a uterus. These systemic failures ultimately lead many people to want hysterectomy.

"His gynecology practice had pictures of babies everywhere, babies, babies, babies, babies, babies." This is how Jackie, a forty-one-year-old white woman working as a pharmacy technician in Tennessee, remembers her doctor's visits in her early thirties. Jackie made frequent trips to this office for several years, desperate for relief from the "gnawing agony" of her unexplained pelvic pain. All the while, in the waiting room, down the halls, and in the exam room, Jackie was surrounded by photos of babies all over the walls—babies that her doctor had delivered. Looking back, she now knows this doctor's office was not equipped to help her, as she wasn't there to get pregnant and give birth but rather to seek diagnosis and treatment for a chronic illness on her ovaries and uterus. As she recalled:

I think that they were not prepared to deal with somebody who was not interested in having kids and who needed help. That was not their department. . . . I wish that they had been kind enough to say, hey, if you don't want kids, and things are going down this road, I would really like you to see somebody else. I wish they had had the guts to say that instead of just letting me come back and back and back and not having any way to help me.

Jackie's doctors never effectively investigated the causes of her pain—which turned out to be endometriosis and ovarian cysts. It wasn't until the media frenzy in 2018 around the actress and director Lena Dunham's hysterectomy for her adenomyosis and endometriosis that Jackie realized she, too, might have an illness and that a surgery could provide relief. After this realization, Jackie found a specialist and got a radical hysterectomy scheduled. This surgery changed her life, or as she says, her hysterectomy "freed" her. "I was actually able to use my brain to do other things than to just block pain," she told me. Yet this freedom, this relief, was put off for most of her thirties because her doctors viewed her symptoms as normal and were not ready to engage in any healthcare that deviated from fertility promotion and birthing. As Jackie recalled:

They were not a hysterectomy kind of place. I think their general bias toward baby factories, or being a baby factory, kept them from being as honest as they could have been. I'm sure that they, like, let me suffer a little bit longer.

Jackie's experience is not unique. In a culture that views pelvic pain as a normal part of "a woman's body" and that centers pregnancy and birth, accessing adequate healthcare can feel impossible. As many interviewees found, hysterectomy seekers must confront a system that views their health concerns as fringe. Though fibroids and endometriosis were discovered in the 1860s,[10] understanding how to identify and treat them is considered "specialized knowledge" that not all gynecologists are equipped with. Similarly, healthcare of trans and nonbinary patients is often deemed a "specialty" that not all doctors are equipped to provide. Amid this system built for cis women having babies, a hysterectomy emerges as a desirable tool of self-care.

HYSTERECTOMY AS A TECHNOFIX

Whether a hysterectomy is chosen to manage one's chronic pain and bleeding, to reduce the risk of future illness, or to forge a new gendered or embodied identity, these various stories point to hysterectomy as a technofix. In an era in which health and well-being are viewed as commodities, and the availability of medical interventions seems endless, many hysterectomy patients understand this procedure as something they can choose to achieve a sense of wellness. Hysterectomy stories exemplify how this surgery has been transformed amid a broader culture in which many of us track our steps, sleep patterns, and heart rate in order to understand ourselves and arrive at or, better yet, "optimize" our health. The next question, then, is who is allowed or able to choose hysterectomy, and what happens when that choice is not freely available?

3

WHO CAN "CHOOSE" HYSTERECTOMY?

Our bodies, ourselves; bodies are maps of power and identity.
—Donna Haraway, *A Cyborg Manifesto*

While there are various reasons for why someone might want a hysterectomy, the freedom to choose this procedure largely hinges on who you are, where you live, and the resources at your disposal. When a hysterectomy is deemed "elective"—as it is in 90 percent of cases—even if it is chosen to manage excruciating pain or bleeding that interferes with daily life, the ability to have the procedure can be limited by doctors, insurance companies, and even hospital policy. As it turns out, this stratified choice is largely due to hysterectomy being caught in the crosshairs of a broader set of reproductive politics. In the absence of adequate funding, research, and training for the various illnesses and conditions affecting the uterus, reproductive politics can take center stage in clinical decisions, as many view hysterectomy primarily as a sterilizing procedure regardless of its benefits. This is because despite the reason for a hysterectomy, there is one absolute that all hysterectomy patients share: becoming sterile or infertile as a result of the surgery.

In simplistic terms, patients are often viewed as choosing between the advantages of a hysterectomy as a mode of self-care and their reproductive capability. As such, choosing hysterectomy is viewed as choosing sterilization, irrespective of its various potential benefits. In particular, choosing hysterectomy often pushes up against the essentialized and constant *potential for motherhood* that people with uteruses often weigh and are weighed down with. The sociologist Miranda Waggoner coined the term *zero trimester* to capture the way women are viewed as "one-day mothers" forever residing in the zero trimester of pregnancy.[1] A close look at hysterectomy experiences builds on this concept by interrogating *which* bodies are construed as existing in the zero trimester and how this concept is unequally wielded across racialized and gendered lines to perpetuate stratified reproduction.

Victoria is someone whose choice to have a hysterectomy is limited by these reproductive politics. She is a twenty-eight-year-old white graduate student working on a master's degree in public policy in New Hampshire. Ever since she was a teenager, Victoria knew she would never want to have children, and this lack of desire has never faltered. Despite this resolution, half a dozen doctors have refused her the option of having a hysterectomy to manage her endometriosis, and she has yet to find a doctor who will green-light her intentions. "It would be one thing if they had all of these health reasons for why it would not be a good idea to get a hysterectomy," she told me. "But instead, I get like, 'Well what if you change your mind about having kids?' And it feels really frustrating and dismissive that I, as a full-grown woman, can't make decisions about my own future and bodily autonomy."

The personal choice for Victoria is clear: she is certain that she wants to opt into the infertility that comes with a hysterectomy in order to alleviate her endometriosis symptoms. Yet she is unable to make this choice happen. As the stories in this chapter illustrate, her inability to make this choice is a symptom of stratified reproduction as her race and gender—specifically, her proximity to white motherhood—are informing the way her doctors make healthcare recommendations. "I had one doctor say, 'You're lucky if you get [a hysterectomy] before you're fifty. We don't do them on young women,'" Victoria recounted to me. "And then she said, 'It would be easier if you were a trans man because then we could just get a letter from a psychiatrist.'"

What Victoria's physician did not mention was the series of hurdles—legal, financial, and logistical—that trans patients who want any form trans healthcare, including hysterectomy, must navigate. In other parts of the country, a trans patient wouldn't have the ease Victoria's doctor is alluding to, as the topography of access to hysterectomy and trans healthcare is complicated across geographic, structural, and legal lines. However, what Victoria's doctor's comments do invoke are the widespread differential policies on hysterectomy based on gender. Frequently, granting a hysterectomy to a young white woman like Victoria, in order to manage her chronic illness, is deemed against a hospital's policy—since she is "too young"—and a doctor will refuse the surgery. For a trans person with the same doctor at the same hospital, and the requisite paperwork, a hysterectomy could be green-lighted, even if they are younger than Victoria. The procedure, of course—and the uterus—remain identical whether the patient is trans or cis, but the reason it is sought is different, as is the gender of the person "housing" the uterus. These external, largely social differences are informing clinical decisions for the same procedure.

As Victoria's story illustrates, having a doctor authorize a hysterectomy is often not based on health reasons alone but on a series of culturally informed medical recommendations that perpetuate long-standing reproductive inequalities. I spoke with Black women who were much younger than Victoria the first time a doctor told them hysterectomy was their only solution for their pain and bleeding. How could it be that even for people with the same symptoms, the necessity of a procedure—and who is deemed "too young" for it—can shift so drastically from person to person?

The hysterectomy stories I collected illustrate how race and gender stratify reproduction as clinicians produce divergent medical pathways for the same procedure. In my interviews with hysterectomy patients—or would-be patients—of various races and genders, I found the following: while white women and nonbinary people tend to have difficulty accessing a wanted hysterectomy, women of color—particularly Black and Afro-Latine women—as well as trans men of all races are often *recommended* a hysterectomy by their provider long before they considered it themselves. Comparing and contrasting these various hysterectomy experiences sheds light on the mechanisms of stratified reproduction and reproductive injustice in a way that involves not only race and class but also trans and nonbinary identities and (dis)ability in the form of chronic illness.

"PREGNANCY IS THE CURE"

The first time Stacey got her period when she was a teenager, it lasted for ninety days. She grew up outside of New York City, and at the age of twenty-four, she still lives in her hometown, where she works as a pharmacy clinician and lives with her longtime boyfriend. Menstruating was always hell—she missed a week of school every single month, as she was essentially bedridden with pain. "I would call my ob-gyn for help, and the nurse would answer," Stacey told me. "She'd be like, 'Sweetie, just take ibuprofen, like, this is normal.'" Six years later, as a college student living an hour away from home, a different doctor finally diagnosed Stacey with endometriosis, a disease she now knows affects 10 percent of people born with a uterus. When Stacey asked her doctor what she could do to make her endometriosis symptoms more livable, he told her that her only options were hysterectomy or a pregnancy, with the caveat that a hysterectomy would likely be inaccessible to her, due to her being "too young" at twenty-one.

Stacey sought a second opinion, and any discussion of hysterectomy was preempted by the doctor telling her she should consider having a baby to cure her endometriosis. Pregnancy as a recommended cure for endometriosis and other reproductive illnesses is not uncommon,[2] as symptoms can abate for some during the pregnancy itself. However, pregnancy is not a panacea. Symptoms typically recur after pregnancy,[3] and pregnancy and childbirth themselves carry significant risk.[4] Moreover, endometriosis, fibroids, and adenomyosis often lead to issues that affect conceiving and sustaining a pregnancy, making this medical recommendation all the more fraught.[5]

"The pregnancy was prioritized for some reason," Stacey told me. "I felt a lot of pressure from the doctors that a hysterectomy was such an extreme choice for me to have at my age." When Stacey explained that she was in college and not interested in having a baby at this time, the doctor explained she did not need to "keep" the baby, but that the pregnancy would be therapeutic in and of itself, thus pushing her to reproduce at any cost, as she relayed in the following account:

> And I was like, I'm not ready to have a kid, what are my other options, and the first doctor was like, hysterectomy—but since you're so young, your insurance may not approve it, you'll have to pay out of pocket. And the second doctor just didn't give it as an option at all. He mentioned children. And he was like, "Well, you could always like, give it up for adoption—you need your body to go through the process to help you." And it's like, even if you give it up for adoption, that's still nine months I'm putting my body through something.

The options Stacey's doctors presented not only were limited but also effectively reduced her from a person seeking a solution for her body's symptoms to a body carrying the potential for creating another life. Neither pregnancy nor hysterectomy seemed fully right for Stacey—she wanted to carry a pregnancy one day, but much later, after she graduated from college and felt settled and ready for parenthood. Yet she subsequently learned about a third option after one of her visits when a nurse told her during intake that she should consider an endometriosis specialist instead of her gynecologist. She took the advice and went on to have excision surgery to physically cut out the endometriosis growths, which significantly reduced the pain. Excision surgery worked for Stacey, and she has had this surgery twice now. She's hopeful she will one day be able to carry a pregnancy to term; if not, she will consider a hysterectomy as a more permanent solution. To this day, she is flabbergasted that a doctor would push her toward pregnancy as a cure for endometriosis. She said, "The option of having a kid at twenty-one didn't seem as extreme to them. That was more prioritized over me being able to get out of bed and have a pain-free day."

It is significant that Stacey is a middle-class white woman, and her story is not reflected across all hysterectomy patients. Primarily white women and many white nonbinary individuals across age-groups in my research were often told they were too young to have a hysterectomy, encouraged to try pregnancy instead as a solution to their chronic illness, or told they must have children first before they could have a hysterectomy. Even in cases where a woman had taken steps to "prove" her convictions about not wanting to reproduce, for example, by having a partner undergo sterilization via vasectomy, this push to preserve a patient's uterus persisted for white participants.

Take Clara, for instance. At the age of twenty-seven, Clara has spent much of her young life in pain, as she's dealt with endometriosis and polycystic ovary syndrome (PCOS) since the age of sixteen. While she believes she has an extraordinarily high pain tolerance, Clara is often forced to call in sick to work as a marketing manager at a company in Utah because she cannot stand up from the pain, and she has had to rush to the emergency room several times following a burst cyst—once for a cyst that was "the size of a mango." Envisioning ways to find relief, Clara has had her heart set since she was twenty on having a hysterectomy, which she believes would greatly improve her quality of life. The oldest of six siblings—whom she essentially raised—she's long been certain that she does not want biological children of her own, and neither does her husband. Also of concern are experiences of the other women in her family with these same conditions who have needed emergency hysterectomies. For Clara, these circumstances combine to both make a hysterectomy feel inevitable and *choosing* it seem optimal.

Yet, despite Clara having no medical contraindications that might prevent the go-ahead for hysterectomy, each of the various doctors she had approached by the time of her interview had refused to perform this procedure for her. One doctor recommended pregnancy itself as a cure for Clara's pain, saying it would provide her with nine "symptom-free" months. But mostly, doctors expressed concern that she was "too young" to close out wanting to gestate a pregnancy and would one day change her mind. Refusing to perform the surgery was framed as a way to prevent this future possibility of regret for her. Clara has tried all sorts of workaround plans. She tried to sign up for a tubal ligation study, thinking if she was already sterilized, the hysterectomy would be green-lighted, but it didn't pan out. Then, her husband had a vasectomy—which took his doctor all of three questions and twenty minutes to agree to—as a way of proving their collective intent to remain childless. Still, doctors declined Clara's request for a hysterectomy. For now, Clara continues to slog through her chronic illness in anticipation of a hysterectomy, while hoping her symptoms don't get worse. Her experiences with doctors have led her to wonder, "Why is my quality of life pulled down? Because you're set on me definitely having a kid one day?"

Jordan offered another such story. Jordan is a twenty-two-year-old white woman living in a beach town in Massachusetts. Her endometriosis and adenomyosis symptoms are so debilitating she can't "conceptualize going to college" and can't work outside of her parents' house, where she lives. Jordan has desperately wanted a hysterectomy to alleviate her symptoms since she was a teenager and is resolute in wanting to be childless, yet she cannot get access to the surgery. Her doctor told Jordan that a hysterectomy is the only option for her adenomyosis, but that he cannot perform it for her due to hospital policy. She told me:

> At this point, the hospital's administration, despite having a disease in my uterus, they just see it as a sterilization option. They do not see it as medically necessary, despite my surgeon specifically telling them that

it was for quality-of-life purposes. No. It won't kill me. It's a benign disease, but I might kill myself because I have it. That's kind of the implication here, and still they denied it.

In her account, Jordan is acutely aware of how a hysterectomy for her is reduced to a sterilization procedure and thus deemed medically unnecessary. Because she is viewed by the healthcare system as "pre-pregnant," her other physical and mental health needs are deemed secondary to maintaining her reproductive capacity.

White women whose ability to sustain a pregnancy was deemed implausible have also nonetheless been blocked from having a hysterectomy. Despite consistent evidence of infertility issues, including that their illness had resulted in so much scarring that a pregnancy would be unlikely, doctors continued to wish to preserve their uterus. One such example is Angelica, a white lesbian living with her wife in suburban Ohio, where she works as an occupational therapist. Angelica says she was open about her sexuality and about her wife, and multiple doctors not only said hysterectomy was her only available treatment option but also told her a viable pregnancy would be nearly impossible for her due to the severity of her endometriosis. Yet Angelica felt her doctors wanted to save her uterus in case a future, hypothetical male partner wanted a child with her. At twenty-four years old she asked for a hysterectomy:

> It was this circular conversation where they said, "You don't have to get rid of your uterus, but you also can never have a baby with it." He kept saying, "What if you change your mind and wanted to be with a man?" And I was like, "I'm never gonna be with a man . . . and having a male partner would not make this medical decision different because you're telling me I will only be safe and healthy if I take it out." They were ready to prioritize fertility over my health, and they were ready to prioritize the possibility of ever having a male partner who would value me for my fertility over my health.

The reasons for denying a hysterectomy for people like Clara and Angelica weren't medical, but rather were rooted in a fear that they would change their mind about their surgery and come to regret this choice. In other words, providers made recommendations based on a fear of anticipatory regret. Others were told they were "too young" to choose such a surgery even well into their late thirties. Instead, they were encouraged to try other routes of treatment for their condition, including various surgeries to remove endometriosis growths and fibroids, as well as treatment with Lupron, an injectable hormone therapy that causes the body to enter a state similar to menopause—whereby in 98 percent of people, loss of menstruation is accompanied by side effects such as hot flashes, decreased libido, depression, and loss of bone density.[6] Their fertility—real for some, but for those who will clearly have infertility issues, imagined—was deemed more important than any other health or quality-of-life concern for which a hysterectomy would be a viable solution. For this group of hysterectomy seekers, their bodies were viewed as residing in the zero trimester, a symbolic or hypothetical temporality in which pregnancy was imagined to be an inevitability that supersedes alternative goals.

While this is the most common experience among the white women I interviewed, variations on this trend were reported by some women of color. One particularly striking example is Carina, a thirty-three-year-old Dominican American woman living with her husband and two kids in Florida, where she runs her own online herbalist shop. Growing up, she was told "bad periods" ran in her family, and for a long time she accepted her extreme, debilitating pain as simply part of her life. When she was twenty-one and living in New York City, however, she was diagnosed with endometriosis. The doctor who diagnosed her then put her through a battery of extensive treatments that many people I spoke to also tried—including ablation surgery (a surgery to burn the endometriosis growths that is now believed to be harmful), Lupron, and Depo-Provera, a contraceptive injection containing the hormone progestin that is administered every ninety days. After none of these worked, the doctor suggested pregnancy. As Carina recalled:

> Then he said, "Well, why don't you try having babies? Because if we do another surgery, it's for me to remove the ovaries and the uterus." I said, "Well, let me just at least try then. Maybe the kids will be the salvation to everything." I thought "Well, all right. I'm married. I guess that's a natural thing to do."

Carina and her husband tried to create a pregnancy "naturally" for a year without success. At around the one-year mark, the doctor told her the endometriosis growths had become bigger, and he strongly recommended IVF, which she and her husband agreed to, and which was quickly successful. Months after she gave birth, she soon realized pregnancy had not cured her illness, and her doctor suggested she try one more time. She recalled:

> I started having pain again and I said, "Oh no, I cannot have pain now with a baby." It was hard enough by myself, now with a baby I can't deal with this. I went back and he was like, "Well, then we will have to do the hysterectomy now." I said OK. Then he said, "Do you have any embryos left?" I said, "Yes, I do have embryos." He's like, "Would you want to use them?" I'm like, "Well, I guess." You know? If this is the only choice I have, I guess I will do that."

Once more, Carina carried a pregnancy in hopes of curing her endometriosis. Afterwards, she found herself with two babies and unchanged symptoms, and decided it was time to have a hysterectomy at the age of twenty-eight. Though the hysterectomy brought immense relief, and she is happy to have her two children, she now regrets not looking into the research or getting a second opinion, and instead just going along with her doctor's recommendations. She told me, "I never did in-depth research—because who was I to question a doctor?"

PUSHING HYSTERECTOMY

As a contrast to being recommended a pregnancy as a cure while being denied hysterectomy, many Black women I interviewed experienced doctors *recommending* a hysterectomy before they ever desired one. This recommendation was often framed as their only choice and frequently verged on coercion. For example, Luna is a Black woman living with her husband in Maryland, where she works for a government agency. Like Stacey, Luna was in her early twenties and had long been experiencing severe endometriosis symptoms, but while Stacey was pushed toward trying pregnancy, Luna was told by her doctor that she *needed* to have a hysterectomy to cure her endometriosis. Both women were college students in large metropolitan areas in their early twenties with severe and debilitating pelvic and menstrual pain later diagnosed as endometriosis. However, Stacey is white, while Luna is a Black woman, leading to drastically different physician interpretations of their age, their fertility, and the implications of a hysterectomy. Luna recalled an ob-gyn appointment she had for her pain:

> They told me that I should get a hysterectomy. And I was like, "I'm twenty . . . ," and then they proceeded to tell me while I was by myself—and they were quite callous about it, very nonchalant. They're like, "You need to get a hysterectomy, you're not gonna be able to have children." And I was like—How are you going to tell twenty-year-old woman that she needs to get a hysterectomy? She can't even drink yet. She hasn't started her life. So I didn't really appreciate that.

Luna finally had a hysterectomy at forty-two after over two decades of ignoring her doctors' suggestions. She tried every alternative she could, but ultimately the pain became too much, and Luna and her husband decided hysterectomy was the right choice.

Tamara, a twenty-nine-year-old Black woman living in Georgia, always envisioned herself one day being pregnant and having children. But her doctors recommended a hysterectomy to her when she was twenty-six years old to manage her symptoms from endometriosis, adenomyosis, and chronic ovarian cysts. She was told there was no alternative. She told me:

> The first time I thought about hysterectomy was when it was presented to me. That's when I seriously thought about it. I knew what a hysterectomy was, obviously, because I'm a nurse and stuff like that, but I never allowed myself to think past that point of "What if I had the hysterectomy." I didn't put myself in that place. I didn't start that process until they said, "You're going to most likely need a hysterectomy."

She and her now husband weighed this recommendation and decided to move forward, and she had a hysterectomy a few weeks later— five days after their wedding. Tamara chose hysterectomy, in a way, not because she wanted it but rather because it was presented as her only choice for relief. Likewise, Daisy, a twenty-eight-year-old Black woman, never considered a hysterectomy for herself until her doctor told her at twenty-seven that it was her only solution for her endometriosis. She recalled:

> He did another exam and he saw that basically my fallopian tubes were shot. My ovary was shot. He was just saying, "I don't see any other way than a hysterectomy." And I trusted him because he's the one that helped me out in the beginning, the one that got me this far. . . . There was nothing left for me to do but a hysterectomy, in his eyes and my eyes.

Like Tamara, Daisy never wanted a hysterectomy, but she wanted relief. When she was told there was no other option, and that a pregnancy was impossible, she agreed to the surgery at age twenty-seven. As the next chapter will reveal, the constrained choice Daisy and Tamara encountered around hysterectomy led to immense grief and feelings of loss.

Kat is yet another person for whom hysterectomy was not only presented repeatedly as an option but who was nearly coerced into having the procedure when she was twenty-eight. Kat is a forty-six-year-old Black woman living in Georgia, where she works in a laboratory as a chemist. Throughout her twenties and thirties, she repeatedly expressed her resolve about having children to her doctors, and her lack of desire to have a hysterectomy. "The doctors would always mention it," she told me. "They first mentioned it to me when I was twenty-eight. And I was like, 'No, I'm not having a hysterectomy at twenty-eight. I want to have children.'" She learned after an excision surgery to treat her endometriosis that her choice had almost been overridden. She was informed by a nurse about a verbal altercation that occurred between her two surgeons while she was under general anesthesia. One of the surgeons was pushing for a hysterectomy, while the other surgeon wished to proceed with the excision surgery as planned. In this retelling, "She was like, 'Just go ahead and do it. She's in pain, she's suffering. Just go ahead and give her a hysterectomy.' He said, 'No, my patient does not want a hysterectomy.'"

Following this revelation, Kat remembered asking herself during an appointment with the aforesaid surgeon, "Why is she pushing a hysterectomy so hard?" Yet this was not an isolated incident by a fringe doctor; providers relentlessly recommended hysterectomy to her throughout her twenties and thirties. As she told me: "Every time I had a physical exam, every time I had a vaginal exam, every time I had a pelvic exam—every time, it was like 'hysterectomy, hysterectomy, hysterectomy.' It was definitely pushed."

While these are individual encounters with individual doctors, together these stories illustrate the disproportionate rate of hysterectomy among Black and brown women. Hysterectomy is often so widespread among women in communities of color that, for some, it comes to be viewed as an inevitable surgery. For instance, Carina, the Dominican American woman discussed earlier, who was told her genetics were responsible for her painful menstruation, recalls only learning how common hysterectomy is in her family when she was set to have the procedure herself:

> When I told my mom, she said, "Oh, a hysterectomy? Yeah. Your aunt so-and-so had it and this other aunt had it," and I'm like, "Wait a minute. What do you mean she had it?" Nobody had told me anything. Why did she have it? She's like, "Oh, yeah. We have bad periods in the family."

Given the stigma surrounding hysterectomy as well as gynecological care more broadly, the pervasiveness of this surgery remains unknown to some, as it was for Carina. In contrast, Hazel, a thirty-nine-year-old Black woman living with her husband in California, where she is a professor of public health, became aware of hysterectomy as an inevitability because her aunt, who, like Hazel, also had endometriosis, had undergone hysterectomy. As she told me:

> I was walking around in grad school in my early twenties, and I said, somebody's going to have to take this out eventually. And I remember that my aunt had a hysterectomy. Certainly no one my age had had it, but I just had this thought. I just remember consciously in my early twenties being like, this is going to go eventually.

This inevitability is rooted in the pervasiveness of hysterectomy as well as the lack of long-term alternatives for many chronic illnesses. Yet as these various stories indicate, a backdrop of racial politics impacts how a doctor might approach a hysterectomy as well as a patients' willingness or reticence to have the surgery.

"NOT USING IT FOR MUCH"

A patient's gender identity also stratifies access to hysterectomy in a way that evokes a trans-specific set of reproductive politics. Many trans patients seeking a hysterectomy did not encounter the concern from their doctors about their age, fertility, or potential regret that many (often white) cis women report. Instead, accessing a hysterectomy was often a relatively easy process as long as they had taken each of the prior steps deemed requisite to their trans medical journey, which generally superseded fertility concerns. These steps typically begin with a gender dysphoria diagnosis and/or letter of approval from a mental health professional and are followed by testosterone therapy, top surgery, and then hysterectomy. Rather than viewing a hysterectomy as a sterilization procedure, then, it is often deemed an obvious next step for trans patients whether they actively want one or not, while many cis women who desperately want the surgery to treat their severe symptoms are discouraged from choosing one.

Consider Sam, a twenty-two-year-old white trans man living in a small city in Alberta, Canada, as a college student who was recommended a hysterectomy when he was nineteen years old. Sam told me:

> I got a hysterectomy about two years ago now and it was kind of mostly because I was in the middle of my gender transition. And it was a suggestion from my doctor, actually. I was sort of asking him in the appointment about birth control, and he said, "Why not just get a hysterectomy? It seems like you don't really need it for much." And I thought, yeah, that's probably true, I probably am not going to use my uterus at all. . . . And it was fairly easy to get access to. So,

I just figured it was the easiest and best decision for me at that point in my transition.

Prior to this suggestion, Sam had not considered a hysterectomy, and it was a low priority compared with taking testosterone and having top surgery, since he no longer menstruated and was not experiencing any pelvic issues. And yet, it was suggested by his doctor in lieu of birth control options, without much questioning of Sam's fertility intentions or discussions of potential regret—even at age nineteen. Meanwhile, many cis women who actively *want* the surgery to treat symptoms that detract from their quality of life—including twenty-two-year old Jordan, described earlier—are forced to undergo dozens of other treatments or simply wait until they're "old enough" before it can be seriously considered.

This quick green light toward hysterectomy was a common experience described by trans men who had "proven" their transness, in a way that was sometimes surprising for the patient. To be sure, accessing each of the prior steps of a routinized trans medical journey is not so simple, as chapter 5 will detail. Many patients must overcome the bureaucratic obstacles of finding trans competent providers and navigate insurance companies that are often ill-equipped to cover gender-affirming care. And yet, the clinician interactions in which a hysterectomy is swiftly approved can be surprising, given the strong emphasis on fertility promotion and preservation for other people with uteruses. For instance, Jake, a biracial (Black and white) thirty-year-old trans man living in New York City and working in book publishing, went to the doctor to discuss the uterine cramping he was suddenly experiencing after years on testosterone. Jake told me he did not expect the ease of getting the surgery approved and the amount of autonomy he was granted in making choices around the surgery—choices like whether to keep his ovaries:

I went in and he was like, "Yes, you are in pain. Do you want a hysterectomy? Like, I'll do it in two weeks." He was like, "You know what you're doing," and I was like, "I do know what I'm doing, thank you so much." And he was like, "OK, I can book you for November 6," which was in two or three weeks. I was like, "OK."

When I asked if the doctor was concerned about Jake's fertility or the possibility of Jake later changing his mind, he explained his doctor's lack of concern as follows:

No, no, because, like, I was already on testosterone. And he was just like, "Do you want your ovaries or not?" And I was like, "I don't know, I'm very on the fence about it." And he was like, "Well, just tell me the day of surgery. And, like, we can figure it out."

In this Jake's account, his doctor not only was *not* using concern of future regret as a way to gatekeep access but also was emphasizing Jake's autonomy in choosing his medical care. Comparing Jake's story with Clara's, for instance, reveals a curious divergence in the clinical understanding of a hysterectomy as a medical treatment. Clara has had debilitating pain caused by her uterus for the much of her life, and yet because she is viewed as one-day pregnant, she cannot choose hysterectomy. Meanwhile, Jake began experiencing uncomfortable cramps for a few months and his doctor immediately suggested a hysterectomy. This difference in clinical approach could be due to a valuing of men and men's pain in clinical spaces—which I've referred to in other work as a patriarchal dividend in medical spheres.[7] Nonetheless, the gender differences in approaches to hysterectomy perpetuate reproductive stratification whereby the degree to which one can choose a hysterectomy hinges on how your body is gendered.

EC is another person who was not expecting such ease in choosing hysterectomy. He is a twenty-eight-year-old white trans man living in a small town in Texas, and he wanted a hysterectomy to ease the dysphoria brought on by menstruation, to permanently eliminate the possibility of pregnancy, and to manage his premenstrual dysphoric disorder (PMDD) symptoms. He explained that after years of trying various forms of birth control, he decided to ask a new doctor for a hysterectomy:

> I went to her like eight months ago, maybe. And just talked to her about what was going on and just told her I've not had good experiences with birth control. I've not had good experiences with the implant, and I'm not interested in running around in circles anymore. And she said, "Well, what would you like to do?" And I said, "Well, I would like a full hysterectomy." So she was like, "You know what, if that's what you want, I trust you and I believe you, and we're going to do it." So that happened in July of this year.

Until only a few months prior to this consultation, EC had identified as a cis woman, and his whole life he has had what he describes as "invalidating" interactions with doctors. This conversation, as a contrast, surprised him. "I was expecting a little bit of resistance," he said, "but she was really just like, 'If that's what you want, then that's what you need.'"

In some cases, these clinical recommendations were guided by a patient having followed the standard steps in trans healthcare, such as those developed by the World Professional Association for Transgender Health (WPATH) or the World Health Organization. Daniel, for instance, a twenty-eight-year-old mixed-race Black man currently living in a large city in England, where he works at a charity, mentioned a straightforward process getting a hysterectomy at twenty-three due to his having followed the routinized prior steps of trans medicine:

> And I managed to get it signed off by a doctor and there wasn't any pushback. . . . I just said, "This is something that I want to do." And

you know, I've had top surgery, I started testosterone when I was sixteen. So I had already kind of gone through the process of kind of going on hormones and getting my first surgery done. So, it wasn't that difficult to get it approved and to get a date in.

In Daniel's case, having already had top surgery and being on testosterone for years justified a hysterectomy as a next step. During such conversations with "little pushback," some mentioned not being fully counseled about fertility preservation or about the permanent sterilization aspect of hysterectomy. Jax, described earlier, for instance, said, "I didn't ever really have conversations about fertility preservation with anyone." Moreover, Jax told me that the sterilization aspect of hysterectomy "was mentioned in the same way as that I would lose my hair taking testosterone." Similarly, Brandon, a twenty-nine-year-old white trans man in Michigan told me, "I would do it again in a heartbeat, and I still don't have any worries that I'm ever going to change my mind." But then he added, "I wish I would've saved some eggs so I could have a kid or something later." For Jax and Brandon, the immense mental health benefits of gender-affirming care, including hysterectomy, make it undoubtedly worth it regardless of side effects or permanent sterilization. And yet, they both acknowledge the lack of counseling on and access to fertility preservation as a source of concern.

Despite these people also having a uterus and the capacity for pregnancy, their stories point to trans people not existing in the zero trimester in the way cis women do. Put differently, trans bodies with uteruses are not construed as inevitably one-day pregnant. While on one hand, the exemption from the zero trimester grants some trans people who *want* a hysterectomy relative access, it can also make the decision either to go forward with hysterectomy or to forgo it a constrained choice. Ultimately, trans patients are choosing hysterectomy in a medical structure that at best forgets about, and at worst devalues or disregards, their reproductive capacity.[8] As an additional constraint, many trans people on testosterone choose hysterectomy as a preventative measure rather than solely for gender affirmation, which the previous chapter detailed, despite a lack of conclusive research on the risk of long-term testosterone therapy. Altogether, the habitual recommendation of hysterectomy to trans patients amid ambiguity about its necessity produces a different reproductive calculus and set of constraints than cis women experience and stratifies reproductive choice based on gender identity.

A key tenet of reproductive justice is the freedom to choose to be a parent. Ushering young trans people to have hysterectomies without full informed consent about their healthcare options, including fertility preservation, is therefore a reproductive injustice. In addition, even if more providers were to have conversations about fertility preservation, such procedures would be out of reach for many given the high cost and complexity of gamete extraction and storage. Gender-affirming care can be very expensive, and many trans patients are forced to crowdsource the money for these procedures; this renders the additional costs of fertility preservation impossible for many.[9] Hence, even when the go-ahead for hysterectomy feels swiftly granted, this choice lies on a continuum between choice and constraint due to a combination of gendered, structural, and biological forces for trans patients.

TRANS ENOUGH?

While the standardized steps of trans healthcare have granted access to those who followed it, they have also been used to gatekeep access to hysterectomy for those who strayed from this medical blueprint. Many nonbinary people I spoke to do not fit into the accepted "trans-normative" idea of a trans patient,[10] whether because they do not experience gender dysphoria in the same way or because they do not wish to undergo testosterone treatment or have top surgery. In the absence of embodying this clear-cut model of transness, which many doctors have come to expect from their trans patients, nonbinary and gender expansive patients are often deemed not "trans enough" for a hysterectomy.

Ocean was in their early twenties when they first asked a doctor for a hysterectomy—though they had yearned for this surgery since they were a teenager. They did not desire taking testosterone or having top surgery and instead prioritized having a hysterectomy for gender-affirming reasons—to no longer menstruate or have the capacity for pregnancy. Despite Ocean being a nonbinary person seeking this procedure for gender-affirming reasons, their doctors were hesitant. Ocean told me, "My first gynecologist said that she was very tied to my uterus—like, 'I don't want you to get it out.' She said something along the lines of uteruses are very important to her." They went on to say, "But, like, I don't understand why you would care about mine. Like, how, I am your client, why are you telling me that you care so much about my uterus?" When I spoke with Ocean, they were twenty-six years old, living in Connecticut with their partner and working as a nursing assistant. Finally able to have a hysterectomy after finding the right doctor who understood their nonbinary identity, they were thrilled to talk about it with me.

Similarly, Arlo, a nonbinary person who has had debilitating endometriosis since age seventeen, sought a hysterectomy at age thirty with a doctor at a woman's clinic. They live in a city in Colorado where they are attending school to be an accountant and have no desire to be pregnant now or any time in the future. Because Arlo did not follow the expected medical steps of masculinization via testosterone therapy and top surgery, they were not viewed by their physicians as a trans person receiving a trans surgery, but rather as a white woman seeking an elective sterilization surgery. Arlo told me the doctor "immediately shut it down and was like, we don't even consider doing that with someone until they've tried every other possible method [for managing endometriosis]." For white nonbinary people like Arlo and Ocean, whose identity does not fit the medicalized, binary notion of transness, their perceived proximity to white womanhood gets in the way of their ability to choose hysterectomy. In the absence of a clear-cut masculine presentation, they are simultaneously viewed as one-day mothers and thus are faced with a "fertility protection" model of healthcare, as well as being invalidated in their gender identity.

Some trans men I spoke to noticed this shift in how doctors treated them and their fertility as they were further into their masculinization journey while taking testosterone. The more they embodied masculinity, the less doctors treated them as pre-pregnant. For instance, Anurag, a twenty-seven-year-old South Asian trans man currently living in Toronto, where he works as a nurse, told me,

> I felt at the time that a lot of when I navigated healthcare as being perceived as a woman consisted of emphasis on fertility that I don't think I really realized. Now I feel that being perceived as male I don't think fertility is ever brought up.

Similarly, Adam, a twenty-seven-year-old Arab trans man, told me, "I was treated poorly up until I started passing as a man. I was treated like shit until I became cis passing." For Adam and others, being gender ambiguous or exhibiting "embodied disruption," as the medical sociologist Emily Allen Paine terms it, led to discrimination and poor healthcare experiences.

Nonbinary patients are often attuned to the valuation of binary identities in healthcare, which, in conjunction with viewing women as pre-pregnant, can make a hysterectomy very difficult to access. One such person is Emmett, a twenty-eight-year-old white nonbinary person pursuing a PhD in geography in West Virginia. Emmett allowed doctors to assume that they were a trans man and that they wanted the surgery for gender affirmation even though they wanted a hysterectomy for chronic issues related to PMDD. Emmett told me, "I think my trans identity helped convince her that I would be a good candidate for surgery, even though I wasn't pursuing the surgery because I am trans," and mentioned not correcting clinicians when they used he/him pronouns due to "bias or confusion around how nonbinary fits into a very binary medicalized system." Since Emmett's PMDD was not taken seriously, they instead had to jump through hoops to "prove" their transness in order to get access to the care they desired:

> I had to get the gender-affirming letters from my psychiatrist and psychologists and a primary care physician and, like, "prove" that I was trans enough. I don't think that I was ever—even in regular consultations prior to surgery—asked what my pronouns were, and I think there was an assumption made that I identify as a trans man. So, he/him pronouns were used consistently. I let them assume I'm a trans man instead of a transmasculine person, because that's something that I know they understand more. It doesn't raise as many questions.

Emmett's experience was invalidation on two levels: their identity as a nonbinary person as well as the severity of their PMDD symptoms calling for a hysterectomy.

There are, once more, exceptions to this trend. One such example is Kai, a twenty-nine-year-old nonbinary person living with their boyfriend in Iowa and working in an administrative role at a university. Kai had been taking testosterone for a few months when they went in to discuss birth control options and remembers being surprised their doctor recommended a hysterectomy:

She said, I want to explain to you all the options you have. And she included the option of hysterectomy and I was probably like, twenty-six or twenty-five. And I was just like, "What? That's an option at this age?" And she said, "Yeah, it's your body, you get to decide what happens." The next day, I was like, I'm ready for this hysterectomy. Let's get this ball rolling.

Despite their surprise when the doctor raised the possibility of hysterectomy, Kai did indeed want the surgery and had one at the age of twenty-seven, all while their doctor affirmed their nonbinary identity and used their preferred pronouns. Clinician competence with nonbinary identities, then, and a patient-centered approach to trans healthcare are key to a positive experience for nonbinary patients like Kai seeking hysterectomy.

FREEDOM TO CHOOSE

When it comes to hysterectomy, reproductive politics based on race and gender impact one's freedom to choose. At its core, choosing hysterectomy is often a decision between the potential benefits of the surgery and maintaining one's potential for pregnancy. As such, many hysterectomy patients are viewed as opting into infertility in order to experience these benefits. And yet, this choice is constrained by a broader set of culturally informed reproductive politics in which choosing hysterectomy is situated. While some bodies are viewed as pre-pregnant, and their fertility is emphasized and paternalistically protected, the reproductive capacity of other bodies is devalued or forgotten about. Specifically, proximity to white motherhood shapes the degree to which a doctor will green-light a hysterectomy. This can make access to a hysterectomy incredibly difficult for white women and many nonbinary people, regardless of their demonstrated desire for the surgery or medical necessity. Meanwhile, women of color and trans men of all races and ages are often steered toward this surgery. Comparing and contrasting the various clinical approaches to hysterectomy reveals the complexity of stratified reproduction, as well as continued reproductive injustices based on both race and gender identity. As it stands, one's freedom to have or not have a uterus, and thus to have or not have reproductive capacity, regardless of if one wants to use it, is limited by how you are perceived by doctors.

4

HOW DO PEOPLE FEEL ABOUT HYSTERECTOMY?

Womb. Gone. Eradicated. You weep for what is lost, but the tears wash nothing away, they just empty you out even further.

—Michelle Sacks, *You Were Made for This*

"It was the best thing I've ever done for my health. Absolutely. No regrets." This is how Lauren explained her feelings about the hysterectomy she had a year prior to our interview. Lauren is a thirty-two-year-old white woman living in Maryland, where she works as a secretary, and is childless. She started asking doctors for a hysterectomy at the age of seventeen, which was met with "alarm" that she would want such a thing as well as the classic retort "you'll change your mind, you're a woman," as she recalls. From the age of twelve, Lauren had menstrual periods that she describes as "intolerable." Until she had the hysterectomy at thirty-one, she was in excruciating pain during every menstrual period, her bleeding was excessive, and having sex was painful.

When I asked Lauren to expound on why a hysterectomy was so great for her, she said, "I have this peace of mind now that I don't have this organ in me that at any point might try to kill me." By "kill me," of course, she means make her life miserable without warning, but nonetheless, removing her uterus removed a huge burden for Laruen.

There are many reasons why someone might willingly opt in to a hysterectomy, and yet these reasons, no matter how solid, are often met with resistance. Many people are told they will one day come to regret this choice and be overcome with grief at the loss of their ability to get pregnant. Others are told they will feel like they've lost symbolic parts of themselves they cannot gain back—feelings of femininity or womanhood, for instance. These assumptions disguised as medical recommendations echo the historical and persistent notion in the cultural imaginary of hysterectomy as an unnecessary surgery that brings only suffering. But how do people who had a hysterectomy actually feel about this choice?

When it comes to all healthcare generally, and even reproductive healthcare specifically, people react in all sorts of ways to the same medical intervention. The reason for undergoing a medical intervention, for instance, can result in different emotional and physical responses. Take the process of IVF, for instance; patients undergoing this regimen to have a child describe it as "painful and emotionally draining," while egg donors undergoing this regimen for a profit describe it as "quick and relatively painless."[1] Even the cultural context in which one lives can shape varying reactions to these supposed biological processes: the physical experience of menopause is perceived differently in the United States, Canada, and Japan, and people report different symptoms altogether.[2] The anthropologist Margaret Lock explains these differences as "local biologies," or time- and place-dependent bodily experiences produced by a dialectic between culture and biology.[3] Given the power of the social and cultural context in shaping medical experiences, it is critical to hear how hysterectomy patients themselves describe how they feel about the surgery and what might be shaping these various reactions.

As I learned throughout my interviews, personal reactions to hysterectomy vary widely—from grief to neutrality to delight. Rather than the hysterectomy itself alone producing feelings of grief or delight, personal reactions to having this surgery largely hinge on the perceived autonomy one has in choosing hysterectomy, and the cultural context in which it is situated.

"I'M A NEW WOMAN WITHOUT OVARIES OR UTERUS"

Samantha is a thirty-six-year-old white lesbian working as a professor in a small town in California, where she lives with her wife. Counter to the common narrative that many women encounter when seeking a hysterectomy (that they will regret it), Samantha says her only regret is not having it sooner. Samantha had to "fight" to have the surgery. She saw dozens of doctors, who told her she was too young or not sick enough for a hysterectomy, and was even forced to undergo a psychological evaluation before a surgeon would agree to the procedure. She finally had the surgery at thirty-two after seven years of debilitating symptoms and begging doctors for relief. She describes her decision to have a hysterectomy as follows:

> It was the best thing I ever did. Oh my god. Yeah. Great. My quality of life has improved like 1,000 percent. I'm very happy that I did it. . . . My only grudge is that like, I didn't, I wasn't able to access it even earlier. My only regret is not being able to get it earlier.

Like Samantha, many women I spoke to were delighted to have had a hysterectomy. This joy surrounding the hysterectomy tended to be particularly tied to the end of menstruation and the alleviation of chronic pain and bleeding. Any feelings around infertility were secondary to the relief and happiness of lessened symptoms. However, these positive feelings of delight, joy, and relief tended to be experienced by those who had to fight for a hysterectomy, which were typically white women. In these cases, hysterectomy patients were actively choosing and desiring a hysterectomy and thus felt empowered once the surgery was finally granted to them.

Echoing Samantha is Janet, a forty-three-year-old white woman working as an administrative assistant and living with her husband and their dogs in Oregon. Like Samantha, Janet is child-free. She told me:

> It was the best thing I ever did for myself was having that surgery. I was a little concerned that it would make me feel less like a woman in some way. But it really hasn't. It hasn't made me feel less feminine or anything and if anything, I feel more confident because I'm not so preoccupied with it. I mean, it served a purpose. And I didn't end up using it for its intended purpose. You know, I was done with it. So, no, it didn't make me feel less feminine or less of a woman.

Many younger white women, regardless of childbearing history, felt similar enthusiasm. Angelica, a white woman in suburban Ohio who had a hysterectomy at twenty-four for fibroids and PCOS said her advice for other women is, "Don't dread it, look forward to it." These accounts of hysterectomy as a source of joy go against accepted cultural messages about hysterectomy as well as prevailing norms within medicine. People who actively choose hysterectomy, whether or not they are childless, can feel relief, happiness, joy, and even more confidence as a result of the procedure.

Women of color who fought for and chose hysterectomy have felt this joy as well. This is because, despite the clear racial patterns both in the ability to choose hysterectomy and in posthysterectomy feelings, the key to a positive hysterectomy experience was feeling agency in choosing to have the procedure. One such person is Faizah, a thirty-one-year-old Black woman living in California, where she works as an administrative assistant at a nonprofit. Faizah had to fight for her hysterectomy in a way that resembled the common struggle among white women. Her symptoms began when she was twenty-six, at which time she started experiencing excessive bleeding during her periods. "I'm talking filling up a tampon and a pad every thirty minutes," she told me. "It wasn't a great way to live, as you can imagine." She went to doctor after doctor to find relief, and none of them seemed to grasp the severity of her symptoms, nor did they try to investigate the cause of this bleeding. Instead, they put her on every type of available contraceptive—every variation of the Pill, IUDs, and shots. "I basically wasted four years of my life going on contraceptives," she said. Eventually, once she was "pretty much bleeding for nine months out of the year," she became set on a hysterectomy. A reluctant surgeon agreed to the hysterectomy after an altercation in his office—during which she bled through her pants onto the doctor's white chair. As the surgeon realized during the surgery, Faizah's symptoms were all along due to undiagnosed endometriosis. After

Faizah's years of struggling, her feelings postoperatively are overwhelmingly positive:

> I honestly can't recommend it enough. I had six years of just pain for what reason? I was not taken seriously, and if somebody had just been like "a hysterectomy might be possible for you" just earlier, like the course of my life would have changed. I'm so excited and happy now. So just in all aspects it got better because of that one, like, three-hour surgery.

Faizah also contradicted another assumption about hysterectomy: that women will feel less feminine after a hysterectomy—an assumption that is amplified in the scant research on women's experience following hysterectomy:

> They say that one of the side effects after the surgery is just sadness because there's like a loss there. I definitely haven't changed anything about me. In fact, like, I have felt *more* feminine after this because I'm not constantly bleeding and feeling disgusting, you know? So yeah, I didn't feel that loss, not for one moment.

Like Faizah, many were pleasantly surprised and relieved after the hysterectomy turned out to be much easier than their doctors' warnings. Yerma, a thirty-seven-year-old, white agender person in New York, is one such person. They desperately wanted a hysterectomy to manage their chronic pain, yet providers repeatedly warned Yerma that the surgery would bring various unbearable symptoms—including chronic anorgasmia (difficulty or inability to orgasm)—none of which Yerma or the majority of hysterectomy patients, typically, experienced.[4] "Doctors told me a lot of horrible things about hysterectomy," Yerma told me, "but for me it was an immediate relief from my symptoms." Despite various warnings from providers, then,

Yerma viewed their hysterectomy as one of the best choices they've made to take care of themselves.

The majority of this group of hysterectomy seekers—those who fought for a hysterectomy and felt postoperative delight—said they did not feel emotionally connected to their uterus and did not experience grief about losing this organ. For instance, Elizabeth is a forty-three-year-old white woman who lives in New York, where she teaches architecture. She had a hysterectomy at age forty-two for fibroids and never had children. She said, "I don't know if it's about being a woman, but I felt like once I had it done, I had my autonomy back. Because all these organs were like conspiring against me for so long that it was just good to be rid of them." Rather than feeling powerless or forced into a hysterectomy, as common assumptions indicate, some people like Elizabeth felt they had their autonomy back because of the surgery.

Stories of posthysterectomy joy also indicate a new way of thinking about one's womanhood as distinct from having organs associated with womanhood. Anabelle, a thirty-one-year-old white woman living in Georgia with her husband and working as an herbalist, had a hysterectomy at age thirty after having had one child. After years of being denied a hysterectomy, she was finally able to have the surgery after signing up for a hysterectomy research study at a university. She said her feelings about her uterus when deciding on the surgery were as follows: "It did what it needed to do. Now I'm not using it and it's only causing problems." Epitomizing this positive spin on hysterectomy and gender was Arizona—a white woman living in a small town in Delaware with her husband. A researcher pursuing a PhD in sociology, Arizona had a hysterectomy at twenty-eight and is childfree. She told me, "I am the best I've been in ages. I am a new woman without ovaries or uterus."

"I FAILED MY ONE JOB"

On the other end of the emotional spectrum, some people certainly felt grief after a hysterectomy. Yet this was typically the case for women who felt pressured by their physician to have a hysterectomy or who were told it was their only option. In these cases, a hysterectomy, and its associated infertility, led to feelings of grief. These negative experiences were most prominent among many Black and Afro-Latine women I spoke to, some of whom said that they fight feelings of being "less of a woman." As such, the same set of reproductive politics that shaped clinician recommendations likewise shape patient reactions to a hysterectomy.

For instance, Tamara, a twenty-nine-year-old Black woman living with her boyfriend in a city in Georgia, where she works as a nurse, had a hysterectomy at twenty-six after years of dealing with endometriosis, adenomyosis, and chronic ovarian cysts. She told me:

> But when the one thing that separates you versus a man is taken away, it makes you question your identity. . . . I struggled with feeling like I wasn't, like, worth being a mom. Or, like, worth being a wife? And when the role that's in question is as deep as being a woman, and whether or not you're good enough to be seen as a woman or good enough to fulfill the role women are supposed to fill and when you ask yourself that, the answer is no, because you don't have a uterus.

Tamara's grief is so strong, she has sticky notes on her mirror to remind herself daily "you are worthy of being a woman" and "you're worthy of being a mom."

The connection between reproducing and womanhood was evident among other women of color in the sample, such as Marisol, a thirty-one-year-old Latina with fibroids and endometriosis who lives in Los Angeles. She refuses to have a hysterectomy because she wants to "have a biological child," but has not been able to carry a pregnancy to full term. She is waiting until she turns thirty-five to have the surgery despite experiencing pain so bad that, as in the story included in chapter 1 in which a woman performed a hysterectomy on herself in the year 1670, she "would want to grab a knife and just literally pull my uterus out of me if I could." The connection for her, between reproducing, her uterus, and her gender identity, comes through in the following account:

> Not being able to have a baby full term almost makes me feel like less of a woman. And I hate that. I hate feeling like I am less of a woman, because I can't carry a child for full term. So, I can only imagine if I didn't have a uterus. I think that would definitely affect my femininity and how I feel as a woman. And it is, you know, it's kinda like a man getting rid of his testicles, you know, or taking out their testosterone. How is a man gonna feel, you know? It's the same.

For Marisol, reproduction and its associated organs are key to her definitions of womanhood. Likewise, Daisy, a twenty-seven-year-old Black woman, echoed these sentiments when I asked how the surgery made her feel about being a woman:

> Oh, I feel like I failed at it. I feel like I failed the one job I was supposed to do. So not being able to reproduce. So I barely feel womanly . . . now I just feel like I'm full male, you know? I know I'm meant for more, of course, but God created woman and man to reproduce. So my job is to reproduce or at least to bring life to the world. And so, I'm not fulfilling my full purpose.

As Daisy alludes to in the phrase "I failed the one job I was supposed to do," some women of color valued their reproductive capacity because of cultural pressures to have babies or, for some, to have large families. For instance, Valeria is a forty-two-year-old Filipino

American woman living in a small city in Texas, where she works at a start-up. She said she regarded her reproduction as a duty to her husband and her family. She had one child, but her endometriosis scarring led to repeated miscarriages, and her pain and bleeding became unbearable. As Valeria recalled, she did not desire a hysterectomy until her mom mentioned it to her:

> My mom told me, "Why don't you just get a hysterectomy? Just get a hysterectomy." And I think that was a permission I needed. You know, because with a lot of immigrant families like, the more—the bigger— the family the better, you know, it was expected that I was going to have like six kids. So, I felt I wanted to hold on to that because I felt like I was letting my husband down and I was letting my family down because I was . . . I was unable to produce . . . reproduce more. And I think that's why I held on to trying that . . . the concept of trying to have a kid for such a long time.

Despite her mom's "permission," Valeria did experience grief— feelings of loss rooted in gendered expectations—after having her surgery at age thirty-nine, saying, "You always associate your uterus with births and reproducing, right? So, yeah, I think for a moment there, I definitely questioned my worth as a woman."

Contrasting accounts like Valeria's with those of women experiencing postoperative joy underscores the diversity of feelings and understandings about the uterus and its removal. For some, their identity as women is not tied to their reproductive capacity or organs, while for others, having their uterus and the capacity for pregnancy is incredibly important. The freedom to choose is key given this variation of feelings. Presuming one will feel overwhelmed with grief, loss, or regret, and thus denying access to the surgery, is simply gatekeeping healthcare based on stereotypes and assumptions. Likewise, failing to consider how a hysterectomy recommendation might make other women, particularly women of color, feel also denies agency and choice. In any case, centering the patient and their particular desires and needs is critical.

As these various stories indicate, it is not only the hysterectomy itself that produces grief but also the broader social context in which a hysterectomy is chosen, and how agentic one feels in choosing hysterectomy. Much as people hold various feelings about what it means to be a woman, or whether one wants to be pregnant or have a family, people can have all sorts of reactions to removing the uterus and what it symbolizes.

SPARK FOR GENDER EUPHORIA—OR INEVITABLE MEDICAL HASSLE?

While delight and gender euphoria were brought about after hysterectomy for some trans men and nonbinary people, many also reported feeling neutral about the surgery. In such cases, a hysterectomy was viewed as one item on a long to-do list in one's medical transition. For instance, Cole is a twenty-one-year-old Black college student and trans man living in California who had a hysterectomy at nineteen. He describes the hysterectomy as a logical next step, and one that was motivated by a desire to mitigate potential risk of exposure to testosterone:

> It was sort of a step in a pretty long process. I had kind of started socially transitioning, kind of at the onset of middle school. And then I had gotten top surgery at fifteen. And then I knew there's like, this kind of ongoing thing in the trans community of like, does testosterone cause like atrophy of reproductive organs? And, for me, it was just kinda like the natural next step. I know, that probably doesn't sound very, like substantial, but it's sort of almost like, logistic wise, it just sort of worked with timing.

Like Cole, many trans and nonbinary interviewees didn't describe gender affirmation as the primary motivator to having a hysterectomy. Instead, as chapter 2 describes in detail, it is often understood as a way to avoid the potential risk of cancer and atrophy—to minimize risk of disease. Accordingly, when it is not viewed primarily as a gender-affirming surgery, having a hysterectomy can elicit more neutral feelings, akin to other "ordinary" health procedures that aren't as culturally contested. For instance, Daniel, a twenty-eight-year-old mixed-race (Black and white) man compared his hysterectomy to another more "neutral" medical procedure said the following:

> I guess I feel quite neutral. It's like, just a necessary medical procedure. . . . Like, if you have like a broken arm, you feel like, "Oh, I'm glad that my arm is no longer broken, I had surgery to fix that," it's kind of like just a neutral feeling.

This neutral feeling was exemplified by Jax's experience. A thirty-two-year-old white man in Chicago who wants a hysterectomy one day, Jax said that for him the surgery is "not very emotional. It seems more practical."

Given the lack of excitement that some trans patients feel about a hysterectomy, the procedure can feel more burdensome than affirming. Jules, a thirty-year-old white trans man living in a small town in Texas, where he works as a professor of sociology, describes a hysterectomy as "a hassle." Accordingly, he hasn't yet had one but plans to, since he feels it would be the responsible thing to do:

> I don't want it enough to overcome obstacles, because it's sort of like getting your flu shot. You know you should get your flu shot, but I'm also not like, excited to get my flu shot, you know, and so if someone makes it really difficult for me to get one, I'm gonna be like, well, screw you. . . . If someone came to me and they're like, I can give you a pill

that will guarantee that you will never get reproductive cancer, I'd be like, OK, I'll do that. And I don't need to deal with this.

In Jules's case, he would much rather avoid a hysterectomy altogether than "overcome" its associated challenges, since he views it as akin to a flu shot—a health procedure you choose due to external pressures to be responsible, but not necessarily one that brings about immediately tangible benefits.

And yet, though many participants weren't anticipating feeling gender euphoria or affirmation as a result of a hysterectomy, gender euphoria came as a happy surprise for some postoperatively. One such person is Harper, a twenty-seven-year-old mixed race (Romani and Native) trans man who works as a barber in Pennsylvania. Harper had a hysterectomy as a requisite step toward an eventual phalloplasty (the surgical construction of a penis). While explaining why he was not particularly enthused about undergoing a hysterectomy, he, like many others, contrasted the benefits of hysterectomy and top surgery:

It wasn't a surgery that I felt like—technically it's a gender-affirming surgery in my case, but it wasn't something that I got to ease any dysphoria. It was more of a means to an end. Top surgery had way more effect on how I physically appeared to other people. And so, like I had a lot of dysphoria around my chest. But I had stopped menstruating as soon as I started testosterone. So aside from the cramping that I'd have every couple of months, I really would kind of forget that I still had the uterus at all.

Despite initially viewing a hysterectomy as a "means to an end," Harper was surprised to feel affirmed as a man after the surgery. As he explained:

The uterus holds so much of like, the concept of womanhood and such, and so to get rid of it, it wasn't something that like I actively thought about beforehand. But afterward, I was like, "Oh, I no longer have the ability to be a mother in that way, you know, at all. I can't get pregnant or anything." And that was like, weirdly, really affirming for me.

As Harper's comments allude, many trans interviewees mentioned having a visceral fear of becoming pregnant prior to the hysterectomy—of "being a mother." Some regarded the thought of pregnancy as "horrifying" or fear-inducing. Because of this fear of pregnancy, even those who didn't necessarily choose hysterectomy for gender-affirming reasons were surprised to feel relief after the surgery when they realized the potential for pregnancy was officially excised. Another such person is Arlo, a thirty-year-old white nonbinary person in Colorado who sought a hysterectomy to deal with endometriosis symptoms. It was only after the surgery that they realized that not having a uterus also affirmed their gender identity: "I just feel more at home in my body and more comfortable knowing that I'm not going to get my period. I'm not going to get pregnant. I'm not going to get cervical cancer because I don't have a cervix anymore." The individual reckonings of a hysterectomy as a gender-affirming surgery are often complex; people simultaneously report deprioritizing a hysterectomy while also expressing gender-related relief after surgery—even feeling more "at home" in one's body after the surgery, as Arlo does.

Moreover, for trans and nonbinary hysterectomy seekers who had to fight for access to the surgery, hysterectomy did spark joy and relief. This is particularly the case for those who, like Arlo, had a chronic illness. For instance, Jeff is a twenty-three-year-old trans man living in California who sought a hysterectomy primarily to manage his severe endometriosis symptoms. Prior to Jeff's transitioning, doctors in his hometown in Virginia rejected his request for a hysterectomy for pain management, but after he moved to California and began his medical transition, a trans health clinic green-lighted the surgery.

Jeff experienced rare but severe postoperative complications with his stitches, which led to two nights in the hospital, yet nonetheless feels overwhelmingly positive. He told me the surgery was "probably the biggest relief I've ever felt in my life." Hysterectomy has freed Jeff from chronic, debilitating pain, from the possibility of pregnancy (which highly distressed him), and from the need to tell employers about his endometriosis symptoms—a conversation that at various times has outed him as trans. As he explained:

> Even the day after my complication, when they were like, "You almost bled to death yesterday," I was like, "That was worth it. I know that my quality of life will be better forever." I did not regret it for one second. Obviously one of the worst experiences I've ever had, but no, absolutely worth it. At no point was I like, "Oh God, I shouldn't have done that or anything." I was like, "That was a terrible complication, but I understand that complications happen."

Those who specifically chose a hysterectomy for gender-affirming reasons also felt postoperative joy. For instance, Aiden is a twenty-nine-year-old white agender person living in California, and a hysterectomy is the only gender-affirming healthcare they desire. When I asked how they felt after the surgery, they said, "I was just ecstatic about it, I was excited. I loved it. Joy, lots of joy even when I was miserable post-op." A primary motivator for Aiden was to remove the possibility of pregnancy, and now that pregnancy is impossible, they are delighted and affirmed in their agender identity. As they told me:

> My peace of mind is incredible. Abortion is no longer a personal issue. It's still an issue that I'm passionate about, but it's no longer a personal concern. This nagging thing that was on my mind was gone. It was a weight off my shoulders, a weight out my abdomen.

For them, the hysterectomy was sought for emotional relief, to affirm their identity through the physical removal of a symbolically gendered organ:

> I remember looking at myself in the mirror after surgery and just, I mean . . . I just felt like myself. I felt a lack of discordance. I felt a change in my sense of self that had moved toward harmony and truth and alignment. I just felt more like me. It's not that I saw it in the mirror—the physical act of looking at myself in the mirror was a materialization of my thought process. And I just . . . I was more *me*.

As these stories highlight, a hysterectomy can elicit various feelings not only preoperatively but also postoperatively. What might begin as a clerical medical procedure can later elicit gender euphoria, particularly as the benefits of removing one's uterus become more tangible. Likewise, while some trans and nonbinary people seeking hysterectomy feel quite neutral, others are delighted and affirmed.

THINKING OUTSIDE THE BOX

In addition to race and gender, sexual orientation has an impact on the way individuals make sense of hysterectomy and the infertility that comes with it. This can be due to different understandings of family and kinship in queer communities. Lesbian respondents, for instance, rarely reported feeling very distressed by their inability to one day be pregnant—the reason being that they had always expected having kids would involve assisted reproduction or adoption. Jamie, a thirty-year-old lesbian and graduate student living in Tennessee, said:

> The combination of being queer, on top of having these sorts of issues, is very strange because I, luckily, don't have a partner who is like, "Why can't we get pregnant?" since you know, getting pregnant would

already be a fucking hassle in the long run, so that's kind of nice know-ing that, that process would be hard either way. So, I'm like, I don't have that pressure, which is good.

The hassle Jamie is referring to is having to use reproductive tech-nologies and sperm donation in order to achieve a pregnancy, which for many queer women across interviews led to a shift in notions of fertility and having kids. The now relatively widespread use of reproductive technologies generally, and among queer people spe-cifically, diminishes the potential for grief or loss associated with a hysterectomy.

Samantha, a twenty-five-year-old white lesbian, described queer reproduction as requiring one to "think outside the box":

> You're not just going to, like, accidentally get pregnant or like start trying and like one day it's going to be an exciting surprise. So you know that it will be something done very intentionally either be-cause you did the research and you save the money and you were able to go through like the adoption system . . . or like in vitro fer-tilization or you found a surrogate or whatever, the amount of plan-ning and expense and all those things you have to brace yourself for in a same-sex relationships. So because you're already thinking outside the box, I do think it informs your opinion of like a family structure and fertility.

These sentiments build on work by the medical sociologist Laura Mamo on queering reproduction, which describes the way lesbians began to use the tools of Fertility Inc.—developed for heterosexual women experiencing infertility—to forge the existence of lesbian reproduction and lesbian families.[5] A decade and a half after Mamo conducted her research, these interviews show queer reproduction to be such an established norm that losing a reproductive organ can be much less distressing or even meaningful for queer women.

The established norm of queer reproduction also shapes how queer women do, and do not, experience compulsory motherhood norms, as Deena a thirty-three-year-old white lesbian, explains:

> I mean, there's certainly not like the pressure from like family members to birth a child. There's no expectation like, even though my wife and I hope to possibly, like adopt or do foster care or something in the future. We don't get the family pressure in the way that my sister-in-law and her husband get like, "Why aren't you guys pregnant yet?"

Due to the acceptance of queer reproduction among lesbians and their families, having a hysterectomy and thus becoming infertile or sterile accrues a different meaning distinct from that for straight women.

Norms around adoption also shaped how many trans and non-binary interviewees make sense of the hysterectomy. For instance, when I asked how it feels to know he can no longer get pregnant after his hysterectomy, Daniel explains:

> If I was a straight trans man, I would feel differently, but kind of my model of family has always been kind of just adopting and like, for long-term relationships, I've always seen myself with a man long term. So, yeah, I've always thought about adopting with like, a male partner. So, you know, I don't feel that strongly about biological kids.

Echoing Daniel, Mac, a twenty-six-year-old white gay trans man attending college in New York City, said simply: "I love kids but just not from my body." Some went one step further to laud adoption as the ideal form of queer family formation. For instance, Stewart, a thirty-four-year-old white bisexual man in Colorado, describes how he felt about children after his hysterectomy:

I did have that thought like, "Oh, now I definitely can't ever have kids." This is the end of that forever, you know, but at the same time, I am also like a really big proponent of adoption. Like . . . I kind of am against people having kids in general. I think there's a lot of kids that need to be adopted first. So, it was not sad for me to be like, Oh, I can't have my own biological kids. I'm like, no, I don't want that.

Similarly, Jeff, a twenty-three-year-old queer white trans man living in rural Virginia, where he works as a barista, echoes the notion of adoption as the ethical—and thus preferred—option that leads to infertility being acceptable and not distressing. (For an in-depth analysis of the adoption industry, I would point readers to the sociologist Gretchen Sisson's book *Relinquished: The Politics of Adoption and the Privilege of American Motherhood*.)[6] As Jeff explained to me:

I honestly think that adoption is far more ethical and just simply a better option. And, so, when doctors were like, "But what if you want to have children?" I'd be like, "If I do want to have children, I already have it worked out but a different thing. That adoption is better for lots of other reasons." So I'm not going to suddenly be like, "But I want to be pregnant."

This trend toward adoption is also due in part to broader notions of family and kinship in queer partnerships. Some respondents mentioned experiencing familial strain due to their identities, which can lead to the salience of "chosen family." Ocean, a twenty-six-year-old nonbinary white person elaborates on this:

For me, my mother and father aren't really family. So it's definitely a found family type of feeling of you know . . . like my friends, you know, those are family. They're like, my real family. So I think adoption just goes along with that idea of found family.

In sum, postoperative feelings about a hysterectomy are shaped not only by gender and race but also by sexual orientation and the accepted queer reproductive and family norms. The norms around assisted reproductive technologies and adoption to create families shape the process of hysterectomy, such that it is not unilaterally a source of grief despite the infertility it brings.

GRAPPLING WITH HYSTERECTOMY'S HISTORY

Hysterectomy's complicated history can also impact how one might feel about this procedure, particularly for patients of color from communities that have been harmed by racialized medical abuse and forced sterilization. For some, this means not choosing a hysterectomy as a rejection of the disproportionate number of hysterectomies performed on Black, Native, Latine, and Chicane women historically and contemporarily. Meanwhile, others find a way to reclaim a hysterectomy and to reframe choosing this surgery as freedom that historically was not always available in their communities.

In other words, even for people whose community has been harmed by sterilization procedures like hysterectomy, the choice is not so clear-cut. The way people discuss choosing hysterectomy echoes work by the anthropologist Iris López on Puerto Rican women in New York City. López found that the long-standing history of forced and coerced hysterectomies and tubal ligations among Puerto Rican women over time led to women themselves *choosing* a sterilization procedure—referred to in Spanish simply as *la operación* (the surgery).[7] Like the women portrayed in López's book, many of the people I spoke to echo the complexity in reproductive health choices for many people of color. While grappling with choosing hysterectomy given its history, people discuss a variety of feelings and reactions, with some finding empowerment in rejecting the surgery, and others reclaiming the ability to choose this surgery. This reveals that, for some, oppressive reproductive technologies can be reclaimed and even celebrated.

One person who long resisted hysterectomy because of its history of racialized abuse is Luna, as recounted in the previous chapter. Luna is a forty-four-year-old Black woman living with her husband in Washington, DC, where she works in public health; a hysterectomy was first recommended to deal with her endometriosis symptoms when she was nineteen. Luna told me that for over two decades, these recommendations were incessant; as she explained, "Every doctor except for one who was also a Black woman told me I should get a hysterectomy." She said she fought these recommendations for as long as she could until, two years prior to our interview, when she was forty-two, because of her knowledge of the long-standing history of racism and anti-Blackness in medicine:

> When it comes to Black women, and communities of color, we've been experimented on since the beginning of this country. You know, the men had Tuskegee and the enslaved women had the gynecologist. To take away the humanity of us being women is real. And it's lasting. It leaves an impression. I mean, the fact that the rates, the maternal mortality rates, for us are unbelievable, and nobody seems to care. There are so many examples of how we don't get taken seriously for our reproductive health.

Similarly, Michelle, a thirty-six-year-old Black woman living with her partner in a small city in North Carolina, where she works at a university, has long suffered from fibroids. While health providers have repeatedly recommended a hysterectomy, and has considered it, her mother had a negative experience with a hysterectomy that she had felt coerced into having. As for Luna, awareness of medical racism and abuse of Black women, coupled with her own mother's history, has led to Michelle delaying a hysterectomy as long as she can. As she explained:

When a hysterectomy is being offered, my questions are: So why are you offering this? Are there alternative solutions? What else would you advise someone else? I am just really aware of what the government has done to control the bodies of Black and brown women. Some people went through forced sterilization. I'm just really acutely aware of those things and I don't distance myself from that at all when speaking with a medical professional.

Lolita, a fifty-seven-year-old Black woman living in a small town in Texas, where she works as a financial adviser, goes one step further to compare hysterectomy rates among Black women to modern-day eugenics. She had a hysterectomy to manage her fibroids at age thirty-six alongside a double oophorectomy. Lolita says she was not properly counseled about the *option* of oophorectomy and the likelihood of surgical menopause. She told me:

It could be a form of population control if the normal procedure for Black women is you don't do anything until the fibroids get so big it causes issues. And then the solution is a hysterectomy. It makes me wonder—is that population control? Is it a form of population control under the umbrella of medicine?

Conversely, others navigate *choosing* a hysterectomy despite these histories. Nicole, a thirty-year-old Black woman in Tennessee who has fibroids and pelvic inflammatory disease, explained the pushback, or stigma, she faces from peers and family members when she mentions her desire for a hysterectomy:

I think that it's jarring for people to witness somebody saying, like, "No, I campaigned for this shit. Like, I wanted a hysterectomy." And knowing that history of hysterectomy is done on Black women, Puerto Rican women, Native women. I think sometimes people have negative feelings about that, because it's like, why would you *choose* to have a hysterectomy? When so many women didn't have? You know, so? And I'm OK with talking about that kind of stuff. But in general, I think folks . . . they just don't understand it. . . . I feel like, honor my ancestors by making choices that they didn't have.

As Nicole explains, choosing a hysterectomy can be viewed as a way of honoring ancestors who were unable to make this same choice for themselves, even if this reframing contradicts commonly held community frameworks about hysterectomy. These sentiments are echoed by Hazel, a thirty-nine-year-old Black woman living in California who has fibroids. Hazel posts often about her hysterectomy on Instagram, which she says she does to raise awareness about fibroids and how Black women can choose a hysterectomy, like she did. Hazel explained that she chose a hysterectomy to raise her quality of life and improve her ability to work and have a social life:

> People think of it as something that is done to you rather than something that they choose to do for themselves. To be fair, you don't really hear or see a lot of people who get hysterectomies. But what is more common for Black women is to hear the experience is somebody who ended up having one that didn't get a chance to choose it. So being someone like me, who says, "OK, this is something I chose to do and here's why." You don't see that.

As the accounts of Nicole and Hazel indicate, hysterectomy has been remade by the widening opportunities for women of color to choose health procedures rather than have them chosen for or forced on them. Choosing hysterectomy is therefore stratified in complex ways that intersect with race, gender, and power.

Ironically and counterintuitively, some people I spoke to even mentioned first seeing hysterectomy as a choice they might want after learning of the procedure through the history of forced sterilization. Similarly, others learned of the possibility of hysterectomy following a family member's negative experience with the procedure. In these cases, becoming aware of a hysterectomy in these negative, powerless contexts sparked curiosity about being able to *choose* this procedure themselves. Vik, a thirty-six-year-old mixed-race (Black, Latine, and Native) nonbinary artist living in a large city in Ontario, remembered the first time they began to consider a hysterectomy:

> Looking back now, it had a lot to do with news of hysterectomy and forced sterilizations of Indigenous women. And, so, because like the news exploded with that in the nineties, I had become very aware of the practice and the possibility of this surgical procedure. And I immediately knew that I wanted it. I got my first period when I was twelve. And already I was like, yeah, this really isn't gonna work and I need this thing out. So I would read my encyclopedias and everything and then the internet. And I was like, OK, I can—this is what I want.

For Vik, learning that a surgery exists to remove the uterus and its associated physical processes prompted curiosity and was a source of hope and excitement. As their comment highlights, technologies of violence can be reclaimed and repurposed over time. Even a procedure such as hysterectomy, entangled as it is in histories of forced sterilization and medical exploitation, can be reconstituted as a way of improving one's life or reaching self-actualization.

FREEDOM TO CHOOSE COMPLEX FEELINGS

Assumptions about how a patient will feel after a hysterectomy are often used to inform clinical decisions. Many providers wish to protect a patient from feelings of regret, grief, or loss and thus might bar access to a hysterectomy. Yet the presumption that all hysterectomy patients will feel the same way about the procedure is not reflected in reality. As this chapter has shown, there are various complex reactions to hysterectomy, ranging from joy to grief and other reactions in between. Rather than the surgery itself eliciting the various reactions, the social context surrounding it is key to shaping one's emotional response. In particular, the degree of agency one feels in choosing hysterectomy can determine whether one feels positively about this procedure. Since race and gender stratify the degree of agency one has in choosing hysterectomy, these same demographic characteristics shape one's feelings about the surgery. For those who fought for the surgery in spite of provider resistance—typically the experience of white women—the response is most often delight and celebration about having had a hysterectomy. People who felt that hysterectomy was chosen for them—typically Black women and other women of color—did feel grief and loss. Trans and nonbinary people, for whom a hysterectomy is recommended as a natural next step in a medical journey, felt the most neutral about the surgery, even making comparisons to other neutral medical procedures like fixing a broken arm. Given the complexity of feelings, blocking patients from the ability to freely choose hysterectomy—even if they may come to regret the surgery—infringes on people's bodily autonomy. Amid this pushback, the next chapter examines the strategies hysterectomy seekers must employ in order to gain access.

5

NAVIGATING ACCESS TO HYSTERECTOMY

I wanted to be an ideal patient. And not to be a difficult patient.

This is how Maura, a forty-six-year-old white genderqueer person from the Pacific Northwest, summed up her medical journey as someone who had experienced pain her whole life. Being a good patient, it turns out, can make things convenient for doctors but can be ruinous for patients. It had taken Maura two decades to be diagnosed as having fibroids and polycystic ovarian syndrome and to finally have the hysterectomy that provided permanent relief.

For years, during regular annual physicals, Maura told doctors about having "difficult periods," only to be instructed to "take some Advil," without further examination. Maura never protested, which she attributes to her family's "Catholic upbringing," explaining, "There's a whole mentality of there is some higher authority who knows better than you do, who will tell you how this is going to go and it's not a culture of challenging." One day during graduate school, in 1999, Maura's pain was so bad she couldn't walk, but her doctor suggested she come in for an examination anyway. Determined and without a car, she set off on foot; upon reaching the hospital's lobby, Maura fainted. Her pain, it turned out, came from a cyst "the size of a grapefruit" on her ovary, weighing it down and causing ovarian torsion—a medical emergency in which the ovary is twisted around itself or the fallopian tube, blocking the blood supply. Maura had an emergency oophorectomy, and when she asked the doctor if she could have her uterus removed too, the doctor laughed off her request. "And then I had recurring cysts and pain until, you know, I finally had the full hysterectomy," Maura told me. That was at the end of 2018, when she was in her early forties—nearly two decades and half a lifetime later.

The majority of hysterectomy stories I collected follow an arc similar to Maura's. At first, patients fully trust their doctors as the experts and therefore do not challenge their recommendations. Perhaps they are told their pain is nothing to worry about or are given a recommendation for a new birth control pill to try, and they are sent home. But in nearly every hysterectomy story I collected, a tipping point is reached after a series of these unsatisfying medical encounters. At that point, the "ideal patient," as Maura calls it, is transformed into what I call the rowdy patient: a person who questions, challenges, and fights back against the medical establishment.

In a system where access to relief from diseases of the uterus and ovaries is highly limited and stratified, hysterectomy seekers must learn to navigate a medical establishment seemingly not built for them. Given the various issues within reproductive healthcare, increasing numbers have turned to do-it-yourself and at-home options: home births, self-removals of IUDs,[1] self-managed medication abortion at home,[2] and even cycle tracking to avoid hormonal birth control. Clearly, however, hysterectomy cannot be done safely as a do-it-yourself procedure. Instead, patients must challenge the healthcare system from within to get answers, relief, and treatments. Hysterectomy patients question their doctors' recommendations, turn to the internet and online networks of patients for answers, and enter the clinical space armed with self-sourced medical research and prepared scripts.

A TRADITION OF PASSIVE PATIENTS

The strategies used by hysterectomy patients go against the notion of a passive and compliant patient that is pervasive in medicine. The term we use—*patient*—has etymological roots in the Latin *patiens*, meaning "to suffer," and evokes an unequal power dynamic between an active healthcare provider and an unresisting, prostrate recipient.[3] Nowhere is this power dynamic more evident than in gynecology, where the very cornerstone of the specialty, pelvic exam training, is underpinned by patient acquiescence. In *Feeling Medicine: How the Pelvic Exam Shapes Medical Training*, the medical sociologist Kelly Underman's analysis of the pelvic exam, a senior physician describes how women were recruited and coerced into practical exams and training for medical students who were being taught the pelvic exam at his university in the 1960s:

> [A faculty member] would go down to the public clinic, manually select a woman, say "You're going to come upstairs and teach the pelvic exam." Not "are you?" or "will you?" "You are." He would completely cover the patient with drapes, including the head ... go into the exam room and the students were probing down this anonymous vagina and roll her out.[4]

Similarly, Terri Kapsalis, author of *Public Privates: Performing Gynecology from Both Ends of the Speculum*, describes the ideal patient in gynecology as "one who is compliant, passive, and accepting rather than active and questioning, a composite of proper womanly performance."[5]

Feminists since the 1960s and 1970s have worked to transform the patient-provider interactions in gynecology. The women's health movement in the 1960s and 1970s, for instance, encouraged women to take charge of their healthcare and to learn how their bodies worked—an effort that culminated in the now iconic comprehensive guide *Our Bodies, Ourselves*. The collective that produced this book also developed a document in 1976 for how to perform a pelvic exam in a more respectful, humanizing manner, which directly influenced the development of gynecological teaching associate (GTA) programs. Medical training for pelvic exams now relies on well-paid GTA volunteers who train medical students themselves, rather than doctors using nameless, floating vulvas cloaked in medical drapes.[6]

The patient-provider relationship is still in flux. Medical sociologists have examined the continuous transformation of patients, using terms like *engaged patient,*[7] *empowered patient,*[8] and *consumer patient,*[9] to describe the ways patients push back against established power dynamics. These are predecessors to the rowdy patient, which many hysterectomy patients must become—simultaneously embodying these various attributes of the modern patient in order to access the care they need. Rowdy hysterectomy patients approach their clinical interactions as engaged consumers, and, if necessary, they see their doctors as being replaceable with different, better doctors. They pore over medical journals and crowdsource advice on Reddit and bring their findings to the clinic, where they actively direct their healthcare. Through these strategies, hysterectomy seekers acquire what the medical sociologist Janet Shim calls *cultural health capital*, defined as a "repertoire of cultural skills, verbal and nonverbal competencies, attitudes and behaviors, and interactional styles" that patients deploy in order to receive more optimal healthcare.[10]

More than four decades after the women's health movement, much work remains to make gynecology equitable not only for women but also for gender and sexual minorities and patients of color. Tracing individual hysterectomy histories reveals the considerable work left to do. Yet these stories also demonstrate incredible agency, resilience, and tenacity, showing how communities take charge of their own healthcare and effectively reshape medicine from within.

A ROWDY PATIENT IS BORN: SHEDDING PASSIVITY AND FINDING RELIEF

Celia's journey exemplifies how one sheds previous passivity to become a rowdy patient—a patient who does their homework, advocates for themselves, and will fire you and find a new doctor if needed. Celia is a forty-one-year-old Black woman living with her husband and toddler son in northern Virginia. She grew up in a military family and is still connected to the military today, working as a case manager for service members and families. Though Celia wasn't raised to question experts or authority figures, concerns for her own health and well-being ultimately led her to challenge the doctors she had long trusted.

"Extremely sharp" pelvic pain started for Celia when she was in her early twenties, which her doctors brushed off as a normal part of the menstrual cycle. She accepted that perhaps she simply had bad periods but one day ended up in the emergency ward of the military hospital due to particularly acute abdominal pain. An ultrasound revealed she had a cyst on her ovary, which doctors assured her was "benign" and therefore "nothing to worry about." Benign, in this case, amounted to cancer-free but did not guarantee escape from bouts of intense pain—including during sex—or, as she would later learn, that her fertility would not be affected.

In Celia's early thirties, she and her husband started trying to have a baby together. Years went by without a pregnancy, so they went to a fertility clinic, where Celia's hormone levels were checked and the couple underwent two rounds of IVF. When these efforts ultimately didn't work, the doctors diagnosed Celia with "unexplained infertility." She asked her doctor if the cyst that was found over half a decade prior could be causing her fertility issues; the doctor said it shouldn't be without looking further into it. Celia remembers thinking, "I'm spending thousands of dollars and you still can't tell me anything?" before switching to a different clinic two hours from their house and run by an endocrinologist.

Looking over her records, the first thing this new doctor said during the consultation was "I noticed you have a cyst. Did they ever remove it?" When Celia told him the cyst wasn't removed because it was "benign," he said, "But how would they know if they didn't go in and see? An ultrasound can't tell you anything." This was the first time Celia realized not all doctors are equipped to provide all their patients with the best care. Thinking about the first doctor who found the cyst, she said, "My doctor at the time was extremely good. But the more I look at it now, I'm like, 'You clearly weren't informed.'"

Despite his assessment of her past doctor, Celia's new doctor recommended as a first next step yet another agonizing round of IVF; when that didn't work, they went ahead with surgery. After the surgery to remove the cyst, her new doctor told her, "I've never seen anything like this." The cyst, which had been growing for years, was fully wrapped around one of Celia's fallopian tubes—it had been preventing a pregnancy and causing extreme pain all along—and the only way to remove the cyst was to remove the entire fallopian tube and right ovary. On the drive home from surgery she remembers crying in the car, feeling completely let down by her providers, and asking herself, "Am I ever going to be able to conceive a child? Am I going to be able to have a child?"

This low point was a catalyst for Celia. She realized she needed to be "her own advocate" and do "her own research" if she was ever going to be free of pain, let alone get pregnant. She started Googling her symptoms and remembers thinking, "I know this is endometriosis." She went to yet another doctor, who recommended Lupron—an injectable hormone therapy that causes the body to enter a state similar to menopause.[11] After looking into Lupron, including searching hashtags on Instagram and reading other women's stories, Celia thought, "Oh no, this is a no. No, boy. This is not what I'm going to do." For the first time, Celia thought, "You know what? I don't think this doctor really knows what she's talking about."

She and her husband eventually did have a child together, through a round of IVF using an egg donor. Shortly after her son was born, however, the pain came back—and this time it was worse. Celia went back to Google, and her searches eventually led her to Nancy's Nook, a "learning library" for endometriosis patients started in 2012 by Nancy Petersen, a registered nurse who has endometriosis herself. Celia credits her new pain-free life as a mother of one to this website, saying, "Oh my gosh, if I would've never found them, I don't know where I'd be."

At forty, Celia finally found a doctor with a specialization in endometriosis, vetted by her newfound endometriosis community. She and her new doctor discussed excision surgery—a surgery that physically excises the endometrial growths and which is currently considered the gold standard in treatment options—after Celia read about it on Nancy's Nook. The doctor agreed to this care but told Celia since the disease had gone unchecked for so long, she couldn't know the extent of the damage without doing surgery, and that hysterectomy was an option. Unfortunately, under the laparoscope, Celia's doctor learned her endometriosis had progressed past the point of excision surgery—hysterectomy was the only solution for a pain-free life. The hysterectomy successfully rid Celia of pain and restored her life, for which she is grateful, but she doesn't feel that she fully "chose" the surgery. Rather, decades of medical negligence chose it for her.

Celia lived through a decade and a half of debilitating pelvic pain, rounds of unsuccessful IVF, and the loss of her uterus and both ovaries. By the time she realized the cause of her infertility, her eggs "were no good," and she was unable to carry a biological child. Serious and widespread deficiencies in provider training were the reason this happened to Celia; doctor after doctor failed to diagnose her endometriosis, neglecting even to properly examine her. The medical system in its current state necessitates rowdy patients. Had Celia continued trudging along as a compliant patient who accepted her doctor's assessments, she would have endured further pain, and perhaps would never have been able to carry her pregnancy with her son. It was not her doctors who helped lead Celia to her new life but rather a series of Google searches, a robust online community, and being "her own advocate" by alternately refusing and requesting treatments counter to or in addition to medical advice. This constellation of private and public actions and agitations is the crux of the rowdy patient.

THE INTERNET WILL SEE YOU NOW: ROWDY PATIENT ACTIVATED

Rather than being passive recipients of healthcare who rely on their provider for all information, budding rowdy patients turn to the internet and social media. Through internet deep dives and online patient communities, they discover critical information on diagnosis and treatments, find lists of vetted doctors—as well as doctors to avoid—and learn strategies, tactics, terminology, and phrasing they can use to get better care. Over time, rowdy patients come to increasingly rely on the information they found themselves, and on the advice of newfound online communities. As Jordan, a Massachusetts blogger, told me, "From the get-go, even your doctors are giving you false information. That's why I go so hard-core on my Instagram page and on my blog. Because how else do you know?" Jordan is one of the many rowdy patients who not only goes to the Internet for help but now spends her time sharing information online herself in order to help others struggling with similar issues.

Instead of simply accepting a doctor's assessment of their pain or gender dysphoria as normal, rowdy patients trust their self-knowledge that something in their body is *wrong* and bring community-sourced knowledge into the clinic, effectively shaping their provider's care. "People think doctors are gods. And they're not, they're human beings," Adina, a fifty-five-year-old white woman who works as a project manager in British Columbia, told me. "And I wish women would feel more confident to question their doctors."

"I KNEW BETTER THAN TO CALL MY DOCTOR"

After years of fruitless doctor's visits, the rowdy patient looks for answers on their own and begins to approach their healthcare like an informed consumer—looking up the latest research on treatments and surgeries in the same way one might browse for clothes online. While discussing frustrations with their doctor's refusal to provide a hysterectomy, Ocean stressed, "I am the client!" evoking the language of a business transaction. As part of occupying an informed consumer role, hysterectomy patients do their homework before entering the clinic and are prepared to teach their doctor on topics as basic as symptomology of illness and transgender terminologies to more complex issues like the most cutting-edge treatments or long-term risks of hormone replacement therapy, for instance.

Bringing their own research to the clinic and getting advice from a newfound community was critical for many in obtaining their desired care—from being diagnosed to getting care that is in line with the most current research. "There's a lot that is wrong with social media, but there's also a lot of great," said Anjali, a twenty-eight-year-old South Asian American therapist living in Southern California with her husband and daughter. "The community that I found via South Asian Warriors has been very, very helpful." Anjali found the online community for South Asian people with endometriosis on Instagram, and the group pointed her toward excision surgery to manage her pain.

Likewise, Yerma, a thirty-seven-year-old nonbinary elementary school teacher living in New York City, told me, "The online endometriosis community literally saved my life." For decades, Yerma experienced chronic pain and bleeding that led to extreme symptoms like vomiting at work and fainting on public transit. Doctors told Yerma that a pregnancy would cure their symptoms, but this led to multiple miscarriages and no relief. Yerma had an aha moment in 2018 after stumbling upon an article in *Vogue* written by Lena Dunham—actress, director, and writer—which narrated her experience seeking a hysterectomy for adenomyosis and endometriosis. In the article, Dunham described her symptoms, which sounded very familiar to Yerma, and also included photos by Georgie Wileman—the artist behind *This Is Endometriosis*, a project that documents people living with the illness. Reading this article, Yerma realized that what they were experiencing were *symptoms* and that life didn't need to be this way. This article and these photos were vital in Yerma's journey toward relief, rather than the dozens of doctors they'd seen for decades.

After realizing they probably had endometriosis, Yerma googled "endometriosis" and found Hyster Sisters and Nancy's Nook on

Facebook—two pages with followers in the tens of thousands. Through these online communities, Yerma learned that an ultrasound is not reliable for identifying endometriosis, and that they should advocate for a diagnostic surgery instead, which they ultimately secured upon request. With this diagnosis and the help of those Facebook groups, Yerma was then able to find an endometriosis specialist and access a much-wanted hysterectomy.

Jamie, a thirty-year-old white lesbian working toward a PhD in Tennessee, similarly experienced years of pain without a diagnosis for nearly a decade until a friend told her to join endometriosis pages, where she, like Yerma, learned she needed surgery for a diagnosis. Jamie ended up having this surgery upon her request, which proved critical to accessing subsequent care, including excision surgery— which she likewise learned about in these online groups. Jamie explained being left with a conflict in her thinking about doctors: she has doubts about physicians' ability to care for her but resists invalidating their knowledge. Instead, as she explained, she wishes experiential knowledge was given more credence:

> I'm not saying that doctors aren't knowledgeable, but I do think there are certain things that you can really only understand by having that experience yourself. And personal knowledge is so important for sick people. And people can read medical studies just as well as doctors can and even sometimes do it better. So, I also got a lot of value out of just other people taking their healthcare into their own hands instead of relying on doctors. And I think that was really pivotal for me, because I knew better than to call my doctor to ask, and just do the fucking research myself.

As Jamie describes, patients with long-ignored chronic illness must rely on community networks, alternative streams of knowledge, and doing their own research in order to get "answers." But, ultimately, patients must then bring this knowledge back to the doctor

and shape their care. In other words, in making healthcare decisions, hysterectomy seekers rely on a mix of traditional biomedical
knowledge along with embodied and crowdsourced knowledge.
Hazel, a thirty-nine-year-old Black public health professor in
Southern California, described "partnering" with doctors: "I try
to impart to doctors that I want to partner with you. You are the
healthcare, I am the self-care. Everything I can do to advance my
healing, I'm going to do."

The consumer-like behaviors of rowdy patients, of course, are not
without precedent. Since the late twentieth century, groups united by
a shared bodily condition—from HIV/AIDS to breast cancer—have
increasingly mobilized against the medical system.[12] These groups
have disrupted traditional frameworks of expertise using disparate
social networks, most recently via "Dr. Google," "Dr. YouTube," and
"Dr. Reddit."[13] Confusion, distrust, and misinformation can also proliferate through these channels, as evidenced during the COVID-19
pandemic, when widespread anti-vaccine and anti-masking sentiments were mobilized from the same sources as earlier questioning
and rejection of child vaccination.[14] The ways hysterectomy patients
describe their medical journeys exemplify these broader changes in
the patient-provider dynamic.

Take Stacey, a twenty-four-year-old white woman on Long Island, recounted her experiences convincing her parents to adopt
her "doctor-shopping" strategy she learned online in order to find
a specialist:

> They always said they're not doctors and to trust the doctor . . . they
> weren't ever ones to question what the doctors were telling me. Until
> I saw in the Facebook group where I was, like, I need to go see a spe-
> cialist. Then my parents were, like, "OK. One hundred percent: find
> it." And I really think you just have to advocate for yourself and do
> your own research. I mean, there were many times I think my doctor's
> office thought I was a crazy Google, Wikipedia, WebMD doctor and

coming up with all these facts, but it helps me in the long run, to get actual care that I deserve.

Wading through a medical system to get "actual care that I deserve" means not only entering the clinic armed with the latest research but taking the additional measure of finding the "good doctors" first—doctors willing to work with rowdy patients and who are committed to finding them relief.

"THIS INFORMATION IS COMING FROM MY COMMUNITY"

Similarly, trans patients often encounter physicians who are not knowledgeable about their healthcare or even their identities. "So many doctors are used to just dealing with cis people," said Sam, a twenty-two-year-old white trans man working in marketing in British Columbia. Many interviewees told me about physicians who were unable to answer basic questions about hormone dosage or surgeries, or who demonstrated an overall lack of familiarity with trans identities and healthcare.

Often, following a series of negative experiences with providers, individuals learn to rely on crowdsourced knowledge and utilize this alternative stream of knowledge to shape their own medical care within the formal healthcare system. "This is the information coming from my community," said Callum, a thirty-one-year-old mixed-race (Black and Latino) trans man in California. "It's so much better."

Across interviews, trans men and nonbinary participants described learning about different surgical methods for hysterectomy, possible side effects of taking testosterone, and types of preventative care that can be lifesaving. The rowdy patient brings this information into the clinic and actively influences their treatment plan. Brian, a twenty-three-year-old mixed-race (Asian and white) trans man in New York City, where he is a graduate student, shared some of his findings from online trans health groups:

There's a lot of information that the doctors will not tell you. I found out that if you take testosterone, there's estrogen cream, which is a good thing to know, for trans men who get hysterectomies but do not want to have vaginal atrophy. And then it wouldn't affect their overall goals on testosterone, which I think is pretty cool.

Similarly, Jules, a thirty-year-old white trans man in Texas, said he regularly tells his provider what he needs, due to the clinician's lack of expert knowledge on how to provide healthcare to trans men. Jules offered the following explanation for why he relies on Facebook groups:

Coming [to the clinic] knowing what you need is so important. Like, I'm the one that said, "You should check my testosterone levels in my blood work" to my most recent doctor, because they were just looking at liver panels and cholesterol and things. But I know what your levels need to be, and you don't want them to be too high and you don't want them to be too low and all of this and so I can interpret that. And so being able to say "Hey, you need to do this."

Ari mentions a similar strategy of doing prior research and being equipped with a document, to preclude becoming a compliant patient. He is a thirty-year-old white trans man in a large city in Illinois, where he is a graduate student. As he told me:

I've had a bad history with doctors. And so, knowing that I'm not going to just shut down in front of a doctor or just accept whatever they're saying is right, is something that, I don't really trust myself to do. So, being able to read up about things beforehand, and know what's going on before I go into a consult feels really important.

Due to the ubiquity of subpar trans care in medicine, or "bad doctors," in Ari's words, trans and nonbinary patients come to rely on community-vetted lists of providers to minimize negative experiences. For Todd, a twenty-six-year-old white trans man attending law school in Illinois, social media is "almost always the first place I look for primary care doctors, hormones, and psychiatric stuff." Jax, a white thirty-two-year-old trans man living in a large city in Illinois, explained the importance of trans communities in identifying providers:

> I find the trans community is usually the main referral to doctors. Because you find one person who has had an affirming experience with a provider and then you're like, this is the person I've heard of, and they're the person I'm going to go to because anyone else is a big question mark, and at least I know this person is less of a question mark, in terms of treating patients. So, yeah, that was the way that I found my original provider that I went to was through some web pages.

Community knowledge is critical to receiving high-quality healthcare for many trans patients, including and beyond which providers to contact and what treatments to request or refuse. Jules said he only realized he needed regular Pap smears because of his social media communities: "There's a big health campaign to get trans men to actually get Pap exams." Since trans patients cannot bypass the medical system altogether, they ultimately must shape it from within. In turn, the community urgency to raise awareness on health issues and to provide lists of "good" and "bad" doctors creates and empowers the rowdy patient. Ultimately, being rowdy is critical for trans patients' well-being and survival.

"I CAN SPEAK YOUR LANGUAGE"

In addition to collecting medical information to bring to the clinic and visiting vetted providers, online communities also foster a sense of defiance against the medical establishment. This collective advocacy takes the form of learning the correct "patient script" in order to get the desired care. "Doctors are very dismissive of people who can't come in and speak to doctors in their language," Lee, a twenty-nine-year-old white nonbinary artist in Arizona, explained. "Those online groups offer a lot of that language." This "language" refers not only to being acutely familiar with the various scientific terms and treatments associated with your illness but also being equipped with an arsenal of phrases to advocate for yourself.

Elena, a twenty-four-year-old woman working as a jeweler in Michigan, told me about the phrases she learned in her online endometriosis groups to use in thorny consultations with a physician:

> If they refuse to do certain testing, you have to say something like "I want it noted on my chart that you refuse testing" and they'll do it. I've adopted that kind of attitude of like, you know, "If you're not gonna listen to me. I'll find someone else because I don't need to put up with this." I think this has helped me be able to get better care.

Elena and many other rowdy patients ask for documentation while also informing their providers that they will find a different doctor if they're unwilling to provide the care they seek—combining the informed consumer attitude with language picked up from their communities.

Jackie, a forty-one-year-old white woman working as a pharmacy technician in Tennessee, learned this lesson as well, after years of having her severe endometriosis and ovarian cysts ignored and normalized by her doctor. As she recalled:

> You really do have to push to find a doctor that listens. Their time is so tensely monetized that you can't spend enough time researching who you're going to go to, because you're gonna have fifteen minutes to plead your case. So, you have to go in, I mean, fully fucking prepared. If you can go in with your own medical case history, that's the

best possible way to do it. You can't, they're not going to lead you to a conclusion. You're your own best advocate 100 percent of the time.

Here, Jackie refers to the process of asking for care from a doctor as "pleading your case." In her experience, you not only need to find a "good doctor" but also come to the doctor's office prepared as if partaking in litigation in court in order to get diagnosed and treated.

Part of patients' pleading their case necessitates collecting extensive documentation of their medical history. Some bring heavy stacks of medical records to appointments, and many seem to have a rehearsed elevator pitch describing their symptoms and medical histories. Oftentimes in the beginning of interviews, a person would start to recite this history, and I had to ask them to pause so I could ask my icebreaker, "So, tell me about yourself."

April is one such person. April is a white thirty-year-old woman living in a small town in South Carolina, where she works as a lab technician. She told me about the tool kit she eventually learned from her online endometriosis communities after years and years of negative healthcare experiences—namely, years of misdiagnoses, failures to identify her endometriosis, and multiple refusals for a hysterectomy:

> I made a list of everything I went through. And I felt like that would help them realize that, hey, she's done everything pretty much possible. Maybe we need to go ahead and do the hysterectomy. So that was really helpful. And then I also have my medical records too. And so, if I go to a new gynecologist, for instance, I can take those with me and say, "Hey, this is what I've done. This is my history."

Nicole, a thirty-year-old Black woman in Tennessee, echoes this, saying what she has learned in her online groups, and what she now tells others, is "Know your body and make sure you have everything documented."

Many people I spoke to mentioned that accruing an extensively documented medical history helps them to be taken seriously. "Being so sick for so long gave me credibility," is how Hallie, a twenty-five-year-old white school psychologist in South Carolina, described her journey. "I can say things like 'This isn't right. I've done this before. Do what I'm asking you to do.'" She learned how to direct and challenge her doctors from years of experience, as well as the feeling of empowerment she gained from her online communities. As she told me, "I know the combination of words to say to get you to listen to me."

"I NEED YOU TO EXPLAIN TO THEM THAT I AM IN PAIN"

Women of color report the additional strategy of proving their "worthiness" as a patient. This can take the form of bringing a support person into the clinic—particularly if that support person is a man or white. Valeria, a forty-two-year-old Filipino American in Texas, described receiving substantially better care when her white husband came with her to doctor's appointments:

> I had to start bringing my husband to a lot of my appointments. I said, "I need you to explain to them that I am in pain, that I am unable to get out of bed. I am unable to function." I absolutely felt crazy many, many, many times, but having my husband there being my advocate helped because that's when they started giving me better medication and stuff like that.

Bringing in a support person, as Valeria now does, is a rowdy patient's solution to a key systemic failure that impacts hysterectomy seekers: the deep-seated racial bias in healthcare, particularly for pain management. While some women of color, at appointments by themselves, might be treated as drug seekers or have their pain minimized, their pain is taken seriously when they are accompanied by a support person.

Pain is often perceived and treated differently by providers when the patient is nonwhite, and particularly when they are Black. This is well documented in health research,[15] including findings that Black patients receive less pain medicine for fractures or appendicitis.[16] In a survey of white medical students and residents, half of the sample endorsed beliefs like "Black people's skin is thicker than white people's," which led to rating Black patients' pain tolerance as higher than that of their white counterparts.[17] In other words, for patients of color with chronic pain, the gendered stereotypes that discount women's pain are exacerbated by racialized stereotypes and anti-Blackness—adding a further barrier to receiving high-quality healthcare.

One person who bore the brunt of these dynamics is Faziah, a thirty-one-year-old Black woman in a large city in California, where she works as an administrative assistant. Faziah recounted her experiences with providers as a Black woman with endometriosis: "Every doctor that I went to that I mentioned pain to treated me like a junkie and said basically, 'We're not gonna give you drugs at all.' But I was simply looking for the reason why this pain was happening."

To push back against the established racism in healthcare, many patients of color used a strategy of introducing themselves within the context of their education or career as a way to assert cultural capital. Michelle, a thirty-six-year-old Black woman living in a small city in North Carolina, where she works in university administration, described this strategy:

I now have a prepared script that I use when I talk to doctors. I've noticed and see a physical change, a shift in posture when I begin to tell them where I work or how many degrees I have. Those things have resulted in a physical changing of attitudes when doctors engage with me, so I say I work at a private, a top thirty, predominantly white school and it makes a big difference. When I say what I do there, when

I say my profession, right, like that makes a difference for people. I've had to use it often as a protection for myself. Like, "I need you to know up front who you're dealing with, and I'm going to ask questions."

As Michelle describes, part of being a rowdy patient for women of color entails showcasing aspects of themselves to their provider—their education and/or socioeconomic status, for instance—to challenge what might be surmised based on racial biases. This adds an extra layer of work for women of color, as they have to show providers "who they are" in order to minimize racist experiences. Kendra, a thirty-one-year-old Black woman living in Florida, where she is a policy analyst, has a similar strategy for pushing back against racial biases:

Sitting down in that chair and saying like, "I'm working on a PhD," means something to people. Until you say very clearly or articulate yourself in a way, they talk to you on a different level, for sure. I tell doctors I live in Boca, which is absolutely posturing. I live in Boca because the university is there, not because I have money. I just live next to campus. So, I say I live in Boca, and they ask, "Oh, where in Boca?" I tell them, "Across the street from campus. I'm working on a PhD." Doctors respond to me in an entirely different way for sure.

As these various stories indicate, racialized patients have an additional hurdle to overcome when becoming rowdy patients. In addition to the various strategies all hysterectomy patients ultimately employ, patients of color must also be equipped with scripts and support persons to showcase their "worthiness" as patients and the legitimacy of their health concerns.

"I FELT LIKE I HAD TO USE THOSE WORDS"

Many trans patients must also have a prepared script to "prove" their transness or otherwise their alleged worthiness for getting care. There is an accepted framework of transness in medicine, as the medical sociologist stef shuster describes in their book *Trans Medicine*. Often, the framework of transness emphasizes being "born in the wrong body," which is a simplistic narrative rooted in a binary understanding of gender. Doctors who rely on these generally outdated narratives might expect to hear that a patient knew from childhood that they were the opposite gender or that they always rejected the traditional gendered expectations of their assigned sex at birth. A person's lived experience isn't always so tidy. Some realize their gender identity later on in life, and one's identification with gender can be complicated— not every transmasculine person rejects all elements of femininity, and of course, many trans people identify as nonbinary. Vik, a thirty-six-year-old Black Latine nonbinary person working as an artist in Toronto, explained intentionally using certain language to make their doctor "understand" their need for a hysterectomy:

> I remember saying something like, "Yeah, I want to have a masculine body" in order to, like, make her understand. I had to say things like "masculine" and "male"—like things that don't really fit in my personal understanding of sex and gender. But I felt like I had to use those words. I had to say, "I didn't feel at home in my body." Which is true. But also, my body couldn't feel at home in this binary society. But it felt like I couldn't be too philosophical.

Another example is Prim, a twenty-four-year-old white nonbinary musician and graduate student living in Massachusetts. Already frustrated by the hassle of accessing a hysterectomy itself, navigating this process as a nonbinary person using they/them pronouns became too difficult. To alleviate this burden, Prim let doctors think they were a trans man who used he/him pronouns in order to make the clinical encounters smoother:

> For ease of everything, I was like, I'm going to do the trans guy thing. I also felt like I needed to construct a certain narrative in order to access medical transition and that I needed to say certain things and present a certain way and to be deemed worthy essentially. For example, I didn't talk about how I have always loved wearing dresses . . . instead I talked about how I was in a store as a kid and I liked a blue vest in the boys' section.

Having to prove transness using specific language is indicative of the tension between expert and experiential knowledge. Many trans men are also very aware of this conflict and are troubled by having to describe their gender in rigid language to providers and insurance companies in order to access care. Brian, the twenty-three-year-old trans man mentioned earlier, said the following about having to be "diagnosed" with gender dysphoria in order to access testosterone and a hysterectomy: "I don't know why this is required by insurance. . . . I think we know our bodies more than some guy who's out here writing insurance code."

Similarly, Enrique, a twenty-two-year-old mixed-race (white, Latino) trans man in New York, views the gender dysphoria diagnosis as a way of gatekeeping care:

> Each psychologist does it differently, but in general it acts as a barrier. As a trans person, basically you have to sit in front of a psychiatrist, and the psychiatrist makes the end decision about whether or not you get to transition, and you don't get to make that choice. If the psychiatrist decides that they don't think that you're trans, then you're not able to get medical care.

As Brian and Enrique indicate, there is a dissonance between how trans patients understand their bodies and their gender and how they must present themselves to providers. This directly pits experiential and expert knowledge such that communities must come together to spread information on the "correct" ways to speak to a doctor in order to access gender-affirming care like a hysterectomy.

Semyon, a twenty-nine-year-old white gay trans man in New York, described being aware of the words his doctor wanted to hear, but pushing back on these scripts:

> And she sort of wanted me to say like "I want this for dysphoria reasons." But like I would rather just talk about like, here's the procedure I would like you to do for me like, is this a procedure that you can do? I shouldn't have to say stuff like that like, "I've always wanted this. This will align my gender with my body." I don't believe any of those things. But I'm like, I'll say them if it gets me surgery.

In these interactions with his surgeon, he explained that he wanted to keep his cervix, which is less common. Semyon had learned on Reddit that the cervix can be important for sexual functioning and was sure about this choice. As he explained:

> She really didn't want to leave the cervix. I think she thought that I like was confusing that with like the G spot, and I'm like no I know where all my organs are like I'm very well informed. And like I'm sure about this. When I pushed back and she did agree to do that, she's like, well, like, you know, you're making my job a bit more difficult. I was like, OK, well, fine, like you can have a slightly more difficult job on this.

As Semyon's story suggests, many trans health providers expect a compliant, passive patient who follows an agreed-upon script. Deviating from the agreed-upon language and norms, in turn, can make a doctor's job "more difficult" but ultimately can allow a patient access to the care they want.

WHAT THE ROWDY PATIENT TEACHES US ABOUT THE PATIENT-PROVIDER DYNAMIC

People who had or want an elective hysterectomy are united by stories of struggle. Whether they are seeking the procedure to treat chronic illness or as part of trans healthcare, patients must navigate a medical establishment that does not understand or prioritize their care. Hysterectomy patients must ultimately embody the rowdy patient—one who questions, challenges, and advocates for oneself in direct violation of gendered expectations of a compliant, passive patient. To access a hysterectomy and high-quality care more broadly, the rowdy patient relies on crowdsourced community knowledge, doctor shopping, and scripted language. In the process, rowdy patients acquire cultural health capital,[18] which empowers patients across racial and gendered lines.

Discussions about medical distrust often describe the conflict in binary terms: either a person fully trusts or fully eschews medicine—as in the case of an antivaxxer, for instance. However, it's often more complicated than this, as many people cannot fully bypass the formal healthcare system altogether. To receive diagnoses, hormone therapies, and surgeries, one must interact with formal providers. The rowdy patient therefore uses the medical system as a tool to achieve their health and embodied goals, while entering the clinic equipped with a script, demanding certain types of tests and care, and being willing to "fire" a provider in the pursuit of a "good doctor." For countless hysterectomy seekers, being rowdy, and viewing themselves and their communities as the experts on their own bodies, proves lifesaving—allowing them to attain a higher quality of life and reclaim their agency after years of needless pain.

CONCLUSION

IMAGINING A WORLD IN WHICH HYSTERECTOMY IS CHOOSABLE

To read about hysterectomy in the news is to read about disaster: emergency hysterectomy after a denied abortion, deadly hysterectomies during war, coerced hysterectomies on detained migrants. A hysterectomy often signals multifold systemic and legal failures, which are then forever written on the body—a body forever changed. Hysterectomy also often indicates a tragedy inflicted by external, malignant forces. Yet one in five people who are born with a uterus will have it removed by the time they are in their sixties, a statistic that was one in *three* when I began this project and one which never ceases to shock the person who asks why I study hysterectomy. With this book, drawing on a hundred stories from people directly impacted by hysterectomy, I sought to figure out what I viewed as a fundamental contradiction: hysterectomy is at once highly common and yet primarily discussed—if at all—as a devastating event that happens *to* you.

By hearing from hysterectomy seekers themselves and delving into the history of this procedure, the story of hysterectomy grows more complicated. While we rarely read about this in news headlines, many people want a hysterectomy, choose a hysterectomy, and are happy to have had a hysterectomy. As my interviewees explained, people might want a hysterectomy for a number of reasons, whether to find freedom from one of the many illnesses that affect the uterus and ovaries or to affirm their gender. These stories contradict fundamental assumptions we hold not only about hysterectomy but about gender, bodies, and reproduction. A pervasive idea within culture and medicine alike is that all people with uteruses will inevitably want to become pregnant and be mothers. Following this logic, choosing hysterectomy will almost certainly spark regret. And yet, as I found, a hysterectomy can elicit various emotional responses, ranging from delight to grief to something in between. While the assumption is that hysterectomy invariably causes grief, it is not the procedure itself that brings on this grief but rather the degree of agency afforded and the social context in which the hysterectomy is situated—the degree to which a hysterectomy feels choosable.

The hysterectomy stories in this book lay bare, in my interviewees' own words, the dangers of viewing "women's bodies" as perpetually pre-pregnant, or as existing in the zero trimester of pregnancy, as the sociologist Miranda Waggoner aptly named it.[1] As it turns out, this ideology can be used within medicine to prevent people from making informed decisions about their bodies, both in the realm of hysterectomy and far beyond. Even opting out of one pregnancy, as in the case of abortion, contradicts central truths we hold about gender in general and women specifically. The abortion scholar Anuradha Kumar and colleagues theorized that abortion is so widely stigmatized because it violates cherished feminine virtues: perpetual fecundity, the inevitability of motherhood, and instinctive nurturing.[2] As an abortion scholar myself, the more I delved into the puzzle of hysterectomy, the more I realized the notion of choosing hysterectomy likewise causes fissures in how our culture understands gender and bodies, perhaps even to a magnified extent. If women are valued for being perpetually fertile, one-day mothers, who are born to be nurturing, how could they ever be happy about removing the organ that is purportedly the source of these fundamental attributes? How could it be that some people would willingly have this organ removed to achieve happier, healthier, more self-actualized lives? Hysterectomy seekers must confront these questions and assumptions in their quest toward a hysterectomy.

Ironically, the overemphasis on fertility promotion within health-care simultaneously leads people to desire a hysterectomy while also making this surgery difficult to access for many. The emphasis on fertility is even found in the way we refer to the uterus and ovaries ("reproductive organs") and to the illnesses that affect them ("reproductive illness"), which erases the other functions these organs hold for bodily well-being.[3] This emphasis is reflected in the financialization of healthcare. Only 2 percent of the National Institutes of Health research budget is allocated toward understanding the various illnesses that impact these organs, many of which lead to a hysterectomy. Accordingly, despite how common these conditions are, patients often require seeing a specialist to receive proper diagnosis and treatment after years of neglect—that is, of course, unless the illness is causing fertility issues, in which case, time to diagnosis typically shrinks.[4] Within this system, people whose uterus is causing suffering might eventually come to desire a hysterectomy for themselves as a mode of self-care. Yet, these same people who wish to *choose* hysterectomy might then be told they are not sick enough, are too young, or haven't had enough babies to warrant a hysterectomy. To have a uterus in a medical system built for cis women having babies often means being pushed to want hysterectomy and then being told to wait.

The freedom to choose hysterectomy is endlessly complicated by gendered reproductive politics as well as a healthcare system that does not invest in understanding and treating the uterus beyond its capacity for pregnancy. As we wade into a second Trump presidency, and the looming possibility of a national abortion ban, understanding these reproductive politics becomes more dire. It is my hope that this book's examination of hysterectomy experiences helps map the social and cultural terrain around all reproductive, sexual, and bodily autonomy battles. In the process, a deep dive on hysterectomy sheds light on broader inequalities faced by people with chronic illness, gender expansive people, and racialized communities. By imagining a world in which hysterectomy is truly choosable, we imagine a world where all people have more freedom to live self-determined lives.

UNEQUAL TECHNOLOGIES

When it comes to medical technologies, we have nearly limitless tools at our disposal for safeguarding our health and enhancing our bodies. We live in an era of robot-assisted surgeries, genomic testing, and Ozempic—all of which enable us to live longer, healthier, more culturally defined aesthetic lives. Our ability to freely use these tools, however, is restricted by social positionality and privilege. Nowhere is this more apparent than in reproductive healthcare, within which one's ability to choose any number of tools—whether birth control, egg freezing, tubal ligation, or the like—hinges on who you are and the resources available to you. Whether one wants to enhance or limit their fertility, all reproductive choices are stratified, limited by interlocking systems of oppression based on race, gender, and class. Moreover, reproductive healthcare is also subject to unique moral panics and cultural ideologies that further limit access—especially for treatments that limit or remove one's fertility. Reproductive health is often used as a proxy battle through which to debate broader values around motherhood, gender, families, and bodies in a way that constrains choice for everyone.

Hysterectomy encapsulates the tension between increasing technology and the ability to freely use this technology to make reproductive health choices. Hysterectomy is safer and more technologically refined than ever before in its history: hysterectomy patients today can receive one to three tiny "keyhole" incisions with minimal scarring and rare minor complications, and they can often leave the hospital that same day. Given this ease, it makes sense that a hysterectomy would become desired, particularly if the organ is causing problems. Yet due to widespread cultural ideologies about hysterectomy, the freedom to choose hysterectomy remains out of reach for many.

Despite rarely being analyzed in tandem, the reproductive battles embedded in abortion access and hysterectomy access alike are linked. Like hysterectomy, abortion is a procedure that has undergone immense technological refinement and yet can be highly difficult to choose due to social stigma. Abortion is now an incredibly safe procedure—fourteen times safer than childbirth, in fact, and in the case of medication abortion, safer than common medicines like Tylenol and Viagra.[5] Given technological advancements, abortion can also be as simple as a few clicks on an app and getting pills shipped that can be taken in the comfort of your home.[6] And yet, access to abortion is extremely limited in most of the country, with access hinging on a person's location and socioeconomic status. Telehealth provision has also long been banned in various states, even before *Roe v. Wade* was overturned, rendering easy-to-access medication abortions available only to those in select states.[7] In both hysterectomy and abortion, ideologies surrounding gender and reproduction are used as a cudgel—wedged between increasingly refined technology and the ability for individuals to make health decisions. In the post-*Roe* context, the need to examine how ideology limits healthcare is increasingly urgent.

As the stories in this book highlight, there are two sides of eugenics logic that continue to influence reproductive healthcare and perpetuate stratified reproduction. The word *eugenics* typically conjures in the social imagination practices that limit "socially inadequate" births, for instance, through forced sterilization practices or through the coercive provision of long-acting reversible contraception (LARC) like the IUD or implant (Nexplanon). Yet *promoting* births viewed as socially advantageous, through abortion bans or lack of access to wanted sterilization procedures, for instance, is a key component of eugenics logic and stratified reproduction. This latter aspect of eugenics might even be on the rise, evidenced by the growing pronatalist movement both in the United States and abroad. This movement, which relies on dubious interpretations of demographic data, warns of plummeting birth rates and "demographic collapse" and is backed by prominent tech titans, including Elon Musk. (Musk, for one, has called low birth rates "a much bigger risk to civilization than global warming.")[8] The unequal provision of hysterectomy showcases the dual mechanisms of eugenics and of stratified reproduction, as some people are barred access to hysterectomy while others are ushered toward it, in a way that reflects these notions of socially adequate or inadequate births.

Hysterectomy access is stratified by race and gender, and more specifically by a proximity to white womanhood. Those who embody white womanhood are often paternalistically barred from choosing sterilization, typically due to a physician's concern about anticipatory regret. Simultaneously, women of color—particularly Black women—are often pushed toward hysterectomy and are told it is the only option for relief from their symptoms. Meanwhile, the reproduction of trans and nonbinary patients is often clerically forgotten altogether during clinical conversations about hysterectomy. Trans men as young as nineteen are recommended a hysterectomy as part of their gender-affirming medical journey while a white cis woman might be told she's too young to choose such a "drastic" procedure at the age of thirty-five. Across race and gender lines, the meaning of "medical necessity" for the same procedure shifts, as do concerns around fertility, age, and regret. While individual doctors might not be consciously acting out of malice—and some might even be motivated by a genuine desire to protect their patients—these individual encounters ultimately make up the fibers of stratified reproduction based on race, gender, and class.

To move forward toward a world where hysterectomy is choosable, then, requires viewing all reproductive health choices through the analytical framework afforded by this study of hysterectomy. This analytical framework is rooted in reproductive justice, is trans-inclusive, and accounts for the complex ways race, gender, history, and politics come together to stratify choice. It is imperative to examine not only who is being barred from the right to choose to parent and why but also who is being barred from the right to opt out of parenting—and thus to opt into infertility. These two infringements are inextricable and together form the bedrock of stratified reproduction and reproductive injustice.

WHAT IS A CHOICE?

For those who *choose* hysterectomy to treat their chronic illness, they choose this procedure in an environment where "women's" health is understudied and misunderstood. Questions that arise in the face of these constrained choices are plentiful. Would these individuals still choose—and feel delight over—this procedure if alternative treatments were possible? For those who choose hysterectomy as part of trans healthcare, would they still choose this procedure in a society that adequately researched and understood trans healthcare? Or in one that recognized and valued trans reproduction and families? These questions, while difficult to answer, reveal the necessity of avoiding the binary of agency versus structure in analyses of reproductive health choices. While an individual might feel a sense of agency in choosing, all reproductive health choices occur amid these broader systemic and cultural failures.

The insights from this book are therefore more complicated than merely declaring that all individuals must have agency in choosing a sterilization procedure like hysterectomy through patient-centered care, which I firmly believe. Instead, the stories in these chapters also reveal the need for structural change. It is critical to invest in understanding the illnesses that affect these organs—including endometriosis, fibroids, and adenomyosis. New diagnostic technologies—beyond exploratory surgery—are also long overdue, and every single provider should be trained in identifying the telltale signs of these diseases. A person with classic signs of endometriosis or fibroids should not have to be told they have this disease by a stranger on Instagram, while their doctor insists that their pain and bleeding are normal. Not to mention, the lack of access to affordable healthcare also constrains hysterectomy choices for all—not only for access to care leading up to a hysterectomy but also for access to fertility-preserving technologies like egg freezing for those who desire it. Making hysterectomy choosable thus necessitates an overhaul in the financialization of healthcare, as well as overarching health research agendas and medical training.

At the same time, trans health must also be properly integrated into the healthcare system. We must invest in researching trans health across the life course as well as trans reproduction and push for health insurance coverage for every aspect of trans health across all fifty states. We need federal protections for trans people, their healthcare, and their doctors. Moreover, every provider should be trained to provide satisfactory, affirming care to trans and nonbinary patients rather than making it necessary for patients to engage in medical tourism and crowdsourcing to find a provider and afford care. As I argue throughout this book, trans health is neither new nor unique: people have been using medicine to alter their bodies to match their gender since before we had antibiotics, and these procedures and therapies are habitually used for cis patients. It is not healthcare itself, then, but rather the social and symbolic meanings underpinning it, that subject trans health to moral panics, unequal access, and legal constraints.

The stories of hysterectomy seekers reveal the extent to which the current healthcare system is not designed for every body. The structural changes that would render a hysterectomy truly choosable would likewise make healthcare more equitable beyond this slice of the population—transforming more and more health decisions into real choices.

BRAVE NEW WOMBS

The personal experiences with hysterectomy presented in this book contribute to various conversations about the structural failures that lead to social and health inequality. Yet despite there being so many stories of struggle, there is also hope. While sexism, racism, and cisnormativity continue to constrain people's healthcare and lives, many are growing increasingly attuned to these inequities. In turn, communities that have been ignored or belittled by institutions of power are sparking conversations—with their families and peers and on social media—and in the process are raising awareness of the various injustices that have long gone ignored. On Facebook, Instagram, Reddit, and the like, people are naming and discussing endometriosis and adenomyosis, questioning why fibroids occur disproportionately among Black women, and sharing strategies of resistance and struggle for others with chronic illness or for others seeking gender-affirming care.

These communities are challenging phenomena within healthcare that have long been accepted as natural or normal, from debilitating pelvic pain to higher rates of hysterectomy among women of color, to lack of trans competency among health providers. By naming these various experiences and providing tool kits of resistance to others, these communities are potentially rebuilding the health system from the ground up. It is my hope that these hysterectomy stories shed light on injustices that span beyond an individual's uterus in an individual clinical encounter. These stories show the resilience and strength of community as well as a vision for a future where healthcare is accessible, trans and queer competent, and in tune with the pillars of reproductive justice.

ACKNOWLEDGMENTS

This book would not be possible without the support of incredible mentors, classmates, colleagues, editors, family, and friends. First, I'd like to thank my adviser and dear mentor, Dr. Susan Markens, who nurtured the idea for *Get It Out* when it began as a text message. Thank you for telling me, "Keep thinking . . ." when I suggested other, much less promising research ideas. Thank you for encouraging me—insisting, even—that this idea should be a book. Endless gratitude to my other incredible dissertation committee members, Drs. Lynn Chancer, Mary Clare Lennon, and stef shuster, for providing support and challenging me to be a better writer and thinker. Stef, your support, wisdom, Zoom sessions, phone calls, and your own incredible book, *Trans Medicine*, made this book possible.

I am boundlessly thankful to the University of California, San Francisco's Advancing New Standards in Reproductive Health, a team of unparalleled scholars whose brilliance and dedication to reproductive rights undoubtedly shaped who I am today. From early on in graduate school, I was in awe of this group, and Dr. Katrina Kimport's abortion incubator program opened so many doors for me. I will forever be honored to have been a part of the team as a postdoc and to have graciously been given the time, support, and space to dedicate to this book. Thank you especially to Dr. Ushma Upadhyay, my mentor and champion during this time, who carved out hours every Friday to co-work with me on Zoom to make sure this book got done. Thanks as well to Dr. Antonia Biggs, Dr. Janet Shim, Dr. Diana Green Foster, Dr. Sarah Roberts, and Dr. Dan Grossman for believing in me and in this book.

I'm also grateful for the support of my academic network. Dr. Rene Almeling, thank you for the feedback, mentorship, edits, encouragement, and your own amazing work. Dr. Jennifer Reich, thank you for choosing this book as part of your series; thank you for your edits and support and for thinking through problems with me. Drs. Dana Johnson and Kathleen Broussard, thank you for reading early drafts and for being such wonderful friends to me; I look forward to seeing you at every repro conference. Viktor and Ange, thank you for your encouragement and for making getting a PhD fun. Pat Kinley, thank you for your excellent edits and your support on this book. Carlo Sariego, thank you for reading early drafts and for your support, friendship, and co-parenting of Tuna. Dr. Laura Mamo, thank you for your encouragement, support, your book *Queering Reproduction*, which inspired me so much as a graduate student, and for connecting me with Frances Phillips. Frances, thank you so much for holding my hand through the editing process, for thinking through this book with me, and for all of your support. Ilene Kalish, thank you for believing in this book. To the anonymous reviewers (and one not-so-anonymous, Dr. Miranda Waggoner), I'm incredibly grateful for your time and feedback. Reviewer 2: when I first read your comments, I seethed, but you made this book stronger—thank you.

I would like to thank mis papás Alan and Lilian, mi tía Yahel, mis hermanos Daniela and Alejandro, tíos Bruce and Jacobo, Bobe Pola, and the rest of my primas, primos, tías, tíos, and sobrinitas. Thank you for letting me talk about hysterectomy and abortion at the dinner table and for being my loudest cheerleaders. Los quiero mucho. Thanks are also in order to the wonderfully nonacademic friends and chosen Brooklyn family, who likewise let me rant about reproductive and sexual health topics at inappropriate settings. Thank you especially to Maxie and Laura, the Haha group chat (Mia, Lilly, Manny, Max) Shea and Adrienne, Caro, Emily and Caroline, Ari and Asher, and Jean-Pierre. Your friendship means

ACKNOWLEDGMENTS

so much to me, and I could not do this work without your love and support. Tuna, thank you for napping next to me while I wrote this book and for being literally the cutest mammal on earth.

My late grandfather, Zeide Mute, te quiero y te extraño siempre. Thank you for always being proud and encouraging of me and my work. Gratitude is in order for my Bobe Surche (Sara Sametz), the forever matriarch of the family, whose strength has long inspired me. With everything I accomplish, she is on my mind—the sacrifices she made, the choices she had and didn't have, and my boundless appreciation for who she was and what she did so that I could be who I am today.

Last but certainly not least: my unending gratitude to every person who sat down with me for an interview and shared their stories with me. Your time, generosity, openness, and trust mean the world to me. Thank you as well to everyone who helped me find these one hundred stories—every like, share, repost, and forward was invaluable.

The research for this book was funded by the Society of Family Planning Emerging Scholars Grant, the Woodrow Wilson Dissertation Fellowship in Women's Studies, and the CUNY Graduate Center Dissertation Fellowship. Thank you to these funders for believing in this book and for funding research that seeks to right the wrongs of decades of science that have neglected the uterus and the people who have one.

APPENDIX

DATA AND METHOD

To analyze contemporary hysterectomy experiences, I conducted one hundred in-depth interviews. In-depth interviewing is an ideal method to capture people's feelings, beliefs, motivations, and practices, which other methodologies cannot glean.[1] This is particularly true for understudied topics such as hysterectomy, since there is a dearth of readily available datasets to analyze. These interviews were with individuals who have had, want, or are considering a premenopausal "elective" hysterectomy. As an additional inclusion criterion, I recruited people who either had a chronic "reproductive illness" such as endometriosis or fibroids, to capture the leading reasons for an elective hysterectomy, *or* who were transgender or nonbinary, to include a historically excluded population in reproductive health literature broadly and hysterectomy specifically. I use *trans* or *transgender* as an umbrella term for those whose gender assigned at birth differs from their gender identity and *nonbinary* to refer to those who identify with a gender beyond the categories of man or woman.[2] Some people in my sample identify with only trans or nonbinary, and some identify as both. In addition, while some trans and nonbinary participants also had a chronic illness ($n = 16$), the majority ($n = 30$) did not. The large volume of interviews allowed for comparisons between cis and trans experiences, as well as comparisons by race and ethnicity and sexual orientation.

I employed a multipronged recruitment strategy to identify participants from varying backgrounds. I targeted social media pages organized around chronic reproductive issues (looking for

key terms: *endometriosis, fibroids,* and *adenomyosis*) and transgender interests and health, distributing calls for participants in
these groups after building rapport with the group administrators.
These groups include EndoBlack, Fibroids Project, EndoWarriors,
and various private and public Facebook groups organized around
transgender healthcare. I also relied on snowball sampling.[3] In this
popular sampling method in qualitative projects, a researcher first
invites potential interviewees within their network and then asks
participants to recommend their contacts who fit the research cri-
teria. This creates a growing chain of interviews. Various participants pointed me to friends or relatives or disseminated my digital
recruitment flyer in listservs and online groups. The flyer read,
"Hysterectomies: Let's talk about it!" and invited individuals who
either have a chronic reproductive illness or identify as trans or
nonbinary to participate in a remote interview.

To address concerns regarding my intentions for conducting research, I positioned myself at the beginning of each interview as a
researcher hoping to fill research gaps on hysterectomy seekers, on
people with chronic illness of the "reproductive organs," and on trans
and nonbinary people. In interviews, I asked participants about their
experiences being diagnosed with chronic illness or with seeking
gender-affirming care; their journey toward having a hysterectomy;
their experiences with medical providers; and their attitudes toward
family formation, reproductive technologies, and the sterility/infertil-
ity associated with a hysterectomy.

Interviews lasted an average of fifty-five minutes and were conducted in 2020 over Zoom or phone, recorded using an audio re-
corder, and transcribed into a transcript. Transcripts were coded and
analyzed abductively using Atlas.ti through multiple iterations—first
garnering broad themes and then tracking a more nuanced set of
themes and subthemes.[4] An abductive grounded theory analysis
allows for new theoretical concepts to develop in response to un-
expected findings against a framework of theoretical knowledge.

After developing broad open codes, I employed axial coding to more closely examine the three primary themes explored in this book: hysterectomy as a technofix, stratified pathways to hysterectomy, and challenging the medical system from within.[5] During this more focused round of coding, data were analyzed for discourses related to a desire for a hysterectomy, emotional reactions to having a hysterectomy and to becoming infertile, and what I call "rowdy patient" strategies, or ways of challenging the medical system to access wanted care. All names that appear in this book are pseudonyms—names either chosen by the participant or selected by me—to further ensure confidentiality. All pronouns that appear reflect participants' named pronouns.

As shown in table A.1, the sample consists of 100 participants—46 trans or nonbinary individuals (24 trans men and 22 nonbinary, genderqueer, or agender) and 54 cis women. Of the 100 participants, 57 are white, 22 are Black, 9 are Latine, and 12 have additional racial identities, including Asian American, American Indian, and Middle Eastern. Of the cisgender women, 36 are straight and 16 are lesbian or bisexual. Of the trans or nonbinary group, only 1 identifies as straight. The average age in the sample is thirty-four years and the range is twenty to sixty-two years. Of those with chronic reproductive illness ($n = 70$), 39 have endometriosis, 26 have fibroids, 11 have adenomyosis, 7 have polycystic ovarian syndrome (PCOS), and 2 have premenstrual dysphoric syndrome, with various interviewees having more than one of these diagnoses. In addition, the majority of participants ($n = 71$) had had a hysterectomy by the time of the interview, while 15 cis women and 14 trans or nonbinary participants had not yet had one (but planned to have one); among those who had had the procedure, 17 cis women and 15 trans men or nonbinary people also had a bilateral oophorectomy. Ninety-five participants were based in the United States across various states and regions, while four were based in Canada and one was in England at the time of the interview.

This study took place during the lockdown phase of the COVID-19 pandemic, which limited my fieldwork and interviews to online and phone formats. Although this format may have limited by ability to foster relationships with communities and community members, my research also unexpectedly benefited from the online data collection in a few key ways. First, global social distancing measures granted me the opportunity to reach individuals across geographic areas from my office, widening the scope of my interviewee sample. Second, many participants who would have otherwise been difficult to reach were able to conduct an interview from their homes—between work meetings, during their down time, or with children in other rooms. This granted me access to folks who ordinarily would be unable to participate in research due to work or caretaking constraints. However, there are also limitations, including the possibility that my sample is biased toward individuals who are most comfortable using the internet and making connections or those from particular class backgrounds who *could* work from home during the pandemic. Next, while interview data yield important insight into peoples' beliefs, motivations, and practices, these data are unable to support causal claims or provide descriptive statistics on the population level. However, given the large volume of data collected, I am confident this study nonetheless provides important insight on an understudied phenomenon and fills various key gaps in the research.

These interviews were incredibly helpful in capturing how people make sense of their healthcare experiences and their bodies. Oftentimes, these interviews were people's first opportunity to share their story in depth, and many thanked me afterward for the time and space to reflect and share. When it comes to "taboo" topics such as hysterectomy, menstruation, and infertility, in-depth interviews with a large, diverse sample recruited online are a powerful way to gain new rich insight.

TABLE A.1. SAMPLE DEMOGRAPHICS BY GENDER AND RACE

	Cis Women	Trans Men	Nonbinary	Total
White	30	12	15	57
Black	14	5	3	22
Latine	5	2	2	9
Other	5	5	2	12
Total	54	24	22	100

NOTES

AUTHOR'S NOTE

1 Irene Kwan and Joseph Loze Onwude, "Premenstrual Syndrome," *BMJ Clinical Evidence* 2015:0806.

INTRODUCTION

1 Parveen Parasar, Pinar Ozcan, and Kathryn L. Terry, "Endometriosis: Epidemiology, Diagnosis and Clinical Management," *Current Obstetrics and Gynecology Reports* 6, no. 1 (March 2017): 34–41, https://doi.org/10.1007/s13669-017-0187-1.

2 Krystale E. Littlejohn, *Just Get on the Pill: The Uneven Burden of Reproductive Politics* (Berkeley: University of California Press, 2021).

3 Arlie Hochschild and Anne Machung, *The Second Shift: Working Families and the Revolution at Home* (New York: Penguin, 2012).

4 Kate T. Simms et al., "Historical and Projected Hysterectomy Rates in the USA: Implications for Future Observed Cervical Cancer Rates and Evaluating Prevention Interventions," *Gynecologic Oncology* 158, no. 3 (September 1, 2020): 710–18, https://doi.org/10.1016/j.ygyno.2020.05.030.

5 Tara Manandhar et al., "Prevalence of Hysterectomy among Gynecological Surgeries in a Tertiary Care Hospital," *JNMA: Journal of the Nepal Medical Association* 58, no. 232 (December 2020): 965–70, https://doi.org/10.31729/jnma.5315.

6 Harini R. and Rachel S. Sushma, "Peri-operative Morbidity between Total Laparoscopic Hysterectomy and Abdominal Hysterectomy for Benign Gynecological Disease: A Prospective Comparative Study," *International Journal of Clinical Obstetrics and Gynaecology* 5, no. 1 (2021): 416–19, https://doi.org/10.33545/gynae.2021.v5.i1g.847.

7 Natalie Angier, *Woman: An Intimate Geography* (New York: Anchor Books, 2000).

8 Lise Cloutier-Steele, Mary Anne Wyatt, and Stanley West MD, *Misinformed Consent: Women's Stories about Unnecessary Hysterectomy*, rev. ed. (Chester, NJ: Next Decade, 2003).

9 Rachel P. Maines, *The Technology of Orgasm: "Hysteria," the Vibrator, and Women's Sexual Satisfaction* (Baltimore: John's Hopkins University Press,

2001); Roy Porter, *The Greatest Benefit to Mankind: A Medical History of Humanity* (New York: W. W. Norton, 1998); Cecilia Tasca Mariangela Rapetti, Mauro Giovanni Carta, and Bianca Fadda, "Women and Hysteria in the History of Mental Health," *Clinical Practice and Epidemiology in Mental Health* 8 (October 19, 2012): 110–19, https://doi.org/10.2174/1745017901208010110.

10 Stanley West and Paula Dranov, *The Hysterectomy Hoax: The Truth about Why Many Hysterectomies Are Unnecessary and How to Avoid Them* (Chester, NJ: Next Decade, 2002); Michele Moore and Caroline De Costa, *Do You Really Need Surgery? A Sensible Guide to Hysterectomy and Other Procedures for Women* (New Brunswick, NJ: Rutgers University Press, 2004); Naomi M. Stokes, *The Castrated Woman: What Your Doctor Won't Tell You about Hysterectomy* (London: Franklin Watts, 1986); Vicki Hufnagel, *No More Hysterectomies* (New York: Plume, 1989).

11 Jean Elson, *Am I Still a Woman? Hysterectomy and Gender Identity* (Philadelphia: Temple University Press, 2004).

12 Susan Markens, "The Problematic of 'Experience': A Political and Cultural Critique of PMS," *Gender & Society* 10, no. 1 (1996): 42–58.

13 Margaret Lock and Patricia Kaufert, "Menopause, Local Biologies, and Cultures of Aging," *American Journal of Human Biology* 13, no. 4 (2001): 494–504.

14 Krystale E. Littlejohn, "'It's Those Pills That Are Ruining Me': Gender and the Social Meanings of Hormonal Contraceptive Side Effects," *Gender & Society*, 27, no. 6 (September 23, 2013): 843–63, https://doi.org/10.1177/0891243213504033.

15 Danielle R. Gartner et al., "Integrating Surveillance Data to Estimate Race/Ethnicity-Specific Hysterectomy Inequalities among Reproductive-Aged Women: Who's at Risk?," *Epidemiology* 31, no. 3 (May 2020): 385–92, https://doi.org/10.1097/EDE.0000000000001171.

16 Anthony N. Almazan and Alex S. Keuroghlian, "Association between Gender-Affirming Surgeries and Mental Health Outcomes," *JAMA Surgery* 156, no. 7 (July 1, 2021): 611–18, https://doi.org/10.1001/jamasurg.2021.0952.

17 Susan Stryker, *Transgender History: The Roots of Today's Revolution* (Cypress, CA: Seal Press, 2008).

18 Trans Legislation Tracker, "2023 Anti-trans Bills: Trans Legislation Tracker," accessed July 25, 2023, https://translegislation.com.

19 Sneha Dey and Karen Brooks Harper, "Transgender Texas Kids Are Terrified after Governor Orders That Parents Be Investigated for Child Abuse," *Texas Tribune*, February 28, 2022, www.texastribune.org; Priya Krishnakumar, "Anti-transgender Legislation in 2021: A Record-Breaking Year," *CNN*, April 15, 2021, www.cnn.com.

20 stef m. shuster, "Uncertain Expertise and the Limitations of Clinical Guide-lines in Transgender Healthcare," *Journal of Health and Social Behavior* 57, no. 3 (2016): 319–32.

21 Kemi M. Doll, Stacie B. Dusetzina, and Whitney Robinson, "Trends in Inpatient and Outpatient Hysterectomy and Oophorectomy Rates among Commercially Insured Women in the United States, 2000–2014," *JAMA Surgery* 151, no. 9 (September 1, 2016): 876–77, https://doi.org/10.1001/jamasurg.2016.0804.

22 S. Intidhar Labidi-Galy et al., "High Grade Serous Ovarian Carcinomas Originate in the Fallopian Tube," *Nature Communications* 8 (October 23, 2017): 1093, https://doi.org/10.1038/s41467-017-00962-1.

23 Doll, Dusetzina, and Robinson, "Trends in Inpatient and Outpatient Hysterec-tomy and Oophorectomy Rates," 876–77.

24 Amandeep S. Mahal et al., "Inappropriate Oophorectomy at Time of Benign Premenopausal Hysterectomy," *Menopause* 24, no. 8 (August 1, 2017): 947–53, https://doi.org/10.1097/GME.0000000000000875.

25 World Professional Association for Transgender Health, "Standards of Care for the Health of Transsexual, Transgender, and Gender-Non-Conforming People [7th Version]," (2012), www.wpath.org.

26 "Committee Opinion No. 701 Summary: Choosing the Route of Hysterectomy for Benign Disease," *Obstetrics & Gynecology* 129, no. 6 (June 2017): 1149, https://doi.org/10.1097/AOG.0000000000002108.

27 "Not Your Mother's Hysterectomy: The Benefits of Minimally Invasive Sur-gery," OBGYN CARE (blog), accessed December 8, 2021, www.obgyn-care.net.

28 E. A. Stewart et al., "Epidemiology of Uterine Fibroids: A Systematic Review," *BJOG: An International Journal of Obstetrics and Gynaecology* 124, no. 10 (2017): 1501–12, https://doi.org/10.1111/1471-0528.14640.

29 Elson, *Am I Still a Woman?*; Chelsea Fortin, Christine Hur, and Tommaso Falcone, "Impact of Laparoscopic Hysterectomy on Quality of Life," *Journal of Minimally Invasive Gynecology* 26, no. 2 (February 1, 2019): 219–32, https://doi.org/10.1016/j.jmig.2018.08.019.

30 Whitney R. Robinson et al., "For U.S. Black Women, Shift of Hysterectomy to Outpatient Settings May Have Lagged behind White Women: A Claims-Based Analysis, 2011–2013," *BMC Health Services Research* 17, no. 1 (August 4, 2017): 526, https://doi.org/10.1186/s12913-017-2471-1.

31 World Professional Association for Transgender Health, "Standards of Care."

32 Ian T. Nolan, Christopher J. Kuhner, and Geolani W. Dy, "Demographic and Temporal Trends in Transgender Identities and Gender Confirming Surgery," *Translational Andrology and Urology* 8, no. 3 (June 2019): 184–90, https://doi.

org/10.21037/tau.2019.04.09; Sandy James et al., "The Report of the 2015 U.S. Transgender Survey," 2016, https://ncvc.dspacedirect.org.

33 Katherine Rachlin, Jamison Green, and Emilia Lombardi, "Utilization of Health Care among Female-to-Male Transgender Individuals in the United States," *Journal of Homosexuality* 54, no. 3 (May 14, 2008): 243–58, https://doi.org/10.1080/00918360801982124.

34 stef m. shuster, "Uncertain Expertise and the Limitations of Clinical Guidelines in Transgender Healthcare," *Journal of Health and Social Behavior* 57, no. 3 (2016): 319–32; stef m. shuster, *Trans Medicine: The Emergence and Practice of Treating Gender* (New York: New York University Press, 2021).

35 Ranee Thakar, "Is the Uterus a Sexual Organ? Sexual Function Following Hysterectomy," *Sexual Medicine Reviews* 3, no. 4 (October 2015): 264–78, https://doi.org/10.1002/smrj.59.

36 Larissa Remennick, "Childless in the Land of Imperative Motherhood: Stigma and Coping among Infertile Israeli Women," *Sex Roles* 43, no. 11 (2000): 821–41.

37 Shellee Colen, "With Respect and Feelings: Voices of West Indian Child Care and Domestic Workers in New York City," in *All American Women: Lines That Divide, Ties That Bind*, ed. Johnnetta B. Cole (New York: Free Press, 1986), 46–70; Faye Ginsburg and Rayna Rapp, "The Politics of Reproduction," *Annual Review of Anthropology* 20, no. 1 (1991): 311–43.

38 Lena Dunham, "In Her Own Words: Lena Dunham on Her Decision to Have a Hysterectomy at 31," *Vogue*, February 14, 2018, www.vogue.com.

39 Rachel Treisman, "Whistleblower Alleges 'Medical Neglect,' Questionable Hysterectomies of ICE Detainees," NPR, September 16, 2020, www.npr.org.

40 Kavitha Surana, "Doctors Warned Her Pregnancy Could Kill Her. Then Tennessee Outlawed Abortion," ProPublica, March 14, 2023, www.propublica.org.

41 Adele E. Clarke et al., "Biomedicalization: Technoscientific Transformations of Health, Illness, and US Biomedicine," *American Sociological Review* 68, no. 2 (April 2003): 181.

42 Susan Markens, Carole H. Browner, and H. Mabel Preloran, "Interrogating the Dynamics between Power, Knowledge and Pregnant Bodies in Amniocentesis Decision Making," *Sociology of Health & Illness* 32, no. 1 (2010): 37–56.

43 Jonathan Metzl, "Introduction: Why 'Against Health'?," in *Against Health: How Health Became the New Morality*, edited by Jonathan M. Metzl and Anna Kirkland (New York: New York University Press, 2010), 1–12.

44 Vence L. Bonham, "Race, Ethnicity, and Pain Treatment: Striving to Understand the Causes and Solutions to the Disparities in Pain Treatment," *Journal*

of Law, Medicine & Ethics 29, no. 1 (2001): 52–68, https://doi.org/10.1111/j.1748-720X.2001.tb00039.x.

45 W. P. Dmowski et al., "Changing Trends in the Diagnosis of Endometriosis: A Comparative Study of Women with Pelvic Endometriosis Presenting with Chronic Pelvic Pain or Infertility," *Fertility and Sterility* 67, no. 2 (February 1997): 238–43, https://doi.org/10.1016/S0015-0282(97)81904-8; K. Ballard, K. Lowton, and J. Wright, "What's the Delay? A Qualitative Study of Women's Experiences of Reaching a Diagnosis of Endometriosis," *Fertility and Sterility* 86, no. 5 (November 2006): 1296–301, https://doi.org/10.1016/j.fertnstert.2006.04.054.

46 Georgiann Davis, Jodie M. Dewey, and Erin L. Murphy, "Giving Sex: Deconstructing Intersex and Trans Medicalization Practices," *Gender & Society* 30, no. 3 (2016): 490–514.

47 Miranda Waggoner, *The Zero Trimester: Pre-pregnancy Care and the Politics of Reproductive Risk* (Berkeley: University of California Press, 2017).

48 Phil Brown et al., "Embodied Health Movements: New Approaches to Social Movements in Health," *Sociology of Health & Illness* 26, no. 1 (2004): 50–80, https://doi.org/10.1111/j.1467-9566.2004.00378.x.

49 Steven Epstein, "The Construction of Lay Expertise: AIDS Activism and the Forging of Credibility in the Reform of Clinical Trials," *Science, Technology, & Human Values* 20, no. 4 (1995): 408–37.

50 Kristin Barker, *The Fibromyalgia Story: Medical Authority and Women's Worlds of Pain* (Philadelphia: Temple University Press, 2009).

51 Emma Whelan, "'No One Agrees Except for Those of Us Who Have It': Endometriosis Patients as an Epistemological Community," *Sociology of Health & Illness* 29, no. 7 (2007): 957–82.

52 Dána-Ain Davis, "Obstetric Racism: The Racial Politics of Pregnancy, Labor, and Birthing," *Medical Anthropology* 38, no. 7 (October 3, 2019): 560–73, https://doi.org/10.1080/01459740.2018.1549389.

53 Littlejohn, *Just Get on the Pill*; Emily S. Mann, Ashley L. White, Cynthia Beavin, and Gabrielle Dys, "Foreign Objects in College Bodies: Young Women's Feelings about Long-Acting Reversible Contraception (LARC)," *Women & Health* 60, no. 6 (July 2, 2020): 719–33, https://doi.org/10.1080/03630242.2019.1710891.

54 Chukwudi Onwuachi-Saunders, Que P. Dang, and Jedidah Murray, "Reproductive Rights, Reproductive Justice: Redefining Challenges to Create Optimal Health for All Women," *Journal of Healthcare, Science and the Humanities* 9, no. 1 (2019): 19–31.

55 Loretta Ross and Rickie Solinger, *Reproductive Justice: An Introduction*, vol. 1 (Berkeley: University of California Press, 2017), 8.

56 Littlejohn, *Just Get on the Pill.*

57 Dorothy E. Roberts, *Killing the Black Body: Race, Reproduction, and the Meaning of Liberty* (New York: Vintage, 1999).

58 Arthur Greil, Julia McQuillan, and Kathleen Slauson-Blevins, "The Social Construction of Infertility," *Sociology Compass* 5, no. 8 (2011): 736–46.

59 Janet K. Shim, "Cultural Health Capital: A Theoretical Approach to Understanding Health Care Interactions and the Dynamics of Unequal Treatment," *Journal of Health and Social Behavior* 51, no. 1 (2010): 1–15.

CHAPTER 1. HOW HYSTERECTOMY'S HISTORY SHAPES ITS PRESENT

1 Chris Sutton, "Hysterectomy: A Historical Perspective," *Bailliere's Clinical Obstetrics and Gynaecology* 11, no. 1 (1997): 1–22.

2 Franklin H. Martin, "Vaginal Hysterectomy for Fibroids of the Uterus," *Journal of the American Medical Association* 26, no. 19 (May 9, 1896): 928–33, https://doi.org/10.1001/jama.1896.02430710030002a.

3 Sutton, "Hysterectomy."

4 Sutton.

5 Ephraim McDowell House, "Ephraim McDowell House," ExploreKYHistory, accessed October 9, 2023, https://explorekyhistory.ky.gov.

6 Sutton, "Hysterectomy," 6.

7 Sutton.

8 Sutton, 10.

9 Rene Almeling, *GUYnecology: The Missing Science of Men's Reproductive Health* (Berkeley: University of California Press, 2020), https://doi.org/10.2307/j.ctv1503gto.

10 Deborah Kuhn McGregor, *From Midwives to Medicine: The Birth of American Gynecology* (New Brunswick, NJ: Rutgers University Press, 1998).

11 "Committee Opinion No. 701 Summary."

12 Cara E. Jones, "Wandering Wombs and 'Female Troubles': The Hysterical Origins, Symptoms, and Treatments of Endometriosis," *Women's Studies*, November 9, 2015, 1083–113. https://doi.org/10.1080/00497878.2015.1078212.

13 Edward Jorden, "A Briefe Discourse of a Disease Called the Suffocation of the Mother (London, 1603)," in *Witchcraft and Hysteria in Renaissance England: Edward Jorden and the Mary Glover Case*, ed. Michael MacDonald (New York: Routledge, 1971), 1–25.

14 Jones, "Wandering Wombs and 'Female Troubles.'"

15 Edward Shorter, "Paralysis: The Rise and Fall of a 'Hysterical' Symptom," *Journal of Social History* 19, no. 4 (1986): 549–82.

16 Maines, *Technology of Orgasm*, 8.

17 Jones, "Wandering Wombs and 'Female Troubles.'"

18 Maines, *Technology of Orgasm*.

19 Michel Foucault, *The History of Sexuality: An Introduction* (New York: Vintage Books, 1990).

20 Elaine Showalter, *Hysteries: Hysterical Epidemics and Modern Media*, vol. 2 (New York: Columbia University Press, 1997).

21 Rachel H. Salk, Janet S. Hyde, and Lyn Y. Abramson, "Gender Differences in Depression in Representative National Samples: Meta-analyses of Diagnoses and Symptoms," *Psychological Bulletin* 143, no. 8 (August 2017): 783–822, https://doi.org/10.1037/bul0000102; Xinyu Qian et al., "Sex Differences in Borderline Personality Disorder: A Scoping Review," *PLOS ONE* 17, no. 12 (December 30, 2022): e0279015, https://doi.org/10.1371/journal.pone.0279015; Andrew E. Skodol and Donna S. Bender, "Why Are Women Diagnosed Borderline More Than Men?," *Psychiatric Quarterly* 74, no. 4 (2003): 349–60, https://doi.org/10.1023/a:1026087410516; Tyler J. Torrico et al., "Histrionic Personality Disorder," in StatPearls [Internet] (Treasure Island, FL: StatPearls Publishing, 2024).

22 Ella Shohat, "Lasers for Ladies: Endo Discourse and the Inscriptions of Science," *Camera Obscura: Feminism, Culture, and Media Studies* 10, no. 2 (1992): 57–90.

23 "Endometriosis," *Yale Medicine*, accessed October 20, 2023, www.yalemedicine.org.

24 Daniela Alberico et al., "Potential Benefits of Pregnancy on Endometriosis Symptoms," *European Journal of Obstetrics, Gynecology, and Reproductive Biology* 230 (November 2018): 182–87, https://doi.org/10.1016/j.ejogrb.2018.08.576; Brigitte Leeners et al., "The Effect of Pregnancy on Endometriosis—Facts or Fiction?," *Human Reproduction Update* 24, no. 3 (May 1, 2018): 290–99, https://doi.org/10.1093/humupd/dmy004.

25 Rachel E. Gross, *Vagina Obscura: An Anatomical Voyage* (New York: W. W. Norton, 2022).

26 James J. Purtell, Eli Robins, and Mandel E. Cohen, "Observations on Clinical Aspects of Hysteria: A Quantitative Study of 50 Hysteria Patients and 156 Control Subjects," *Journal of the American Medical Association* 146, no. 10 (1951): 905.

27 International Planned Parenthood Federation, *Client-Centred Clinical Guidelines for Sexual and Reproductive Healthcare*, 2022, www.ippf.org.

28 Indiana Eugenics: History and Legacy (website), accessed October 25, 2023, https://eugenics.iupui.edu/.

29 *Buck v. Bell*, 274 U.S. 200 (1927), Justia Law, accessed October 25, 2023, https://supreme.justia.com/cases/federal/us/274/200/.

30 Alexandra Minna Stern, "Sterilized in the Name of Public Health: Race, Immigration, and Reproductive Control in Modern California," *American Journal of Public Health* 95, no. 7 (2005): 1128–38.

31 Edwin Black, "Hitler's Debt to America," *The Guardian*, February 6, 2004, sec. World News, www.theguardian.com.

32 Alexandra Minna Stern, *Eugenic Nation: Faults and Frontiers of Better Breeding in Modern America* (Berkeley: University of California Press, 2016).

33 Nicole L. Novak et al., "Disproportionate Sterilization of Latinos under California's Eugenic Sterilization Program, 1920–1945," *American Journal of Public Health* 108, no. 5 (2018): 611–13.

34 Natalie Lira and Alexandra Minna Stern, "Mexican Americans and Eugenic Sterilization: Resisting Reproductive Injustice in California, 1920–1950," *Aztlan: A Journal of Chicano Studies* 39, no. 2 (September 1, 2014): 9–34; Vicki L. Ruiz, *From Out of the Shadows: Mexican Women in Twentieth-Century America* (New York: Oxford University Press, 2008).

35 Iris Ofelia López, *Matters of Choice: Puerto Rican Women's Struggle for Reproductive Freedom* (New Brunswick, NJ: Rutgers University Press, 2008).

36 Barbara Gurr, "Mothering in the Borderlands: Policing Native American Women's Reproductive Healthcare," *International Journal of Sociology of the Family* 37, no. 1 (2011): 69–84.

37 Jane Lawrence, "The Indian Health Service and the Sterilization of Native American Women," *American Indian Quarterly* 24, no. 3 (2000): 400–419, https://www.jstor.org/stable/1185911.

38 U.S. Government Accountability Office, "Investigation of Allegations Concerning Indian Health Service," November 4, 1974, www.gao.gov.

39 Zakiya Luna and Kristin Luker, "Reproductive Justice," *Annual Review of Law and Social Science* 9 (2013): 327–52.

40 Laura Briggs, *Reproducing Empire* (Berkeley: University of California Press, 2003), www.ucpress.edu.

41 Laura Briggs, "'The Pill' in Puerto Rico and the Mainland United States: Negotiating Discourses of Risk and Decolonization," in *Governing the Female Body: Gender, Health, and Networks of Power*, ed. Lori Reed and Pamela Saukko (Albany: State University of New York Press, 2010), 159–83.

42 Elena R. Gutiérrez and Liza Fuentes, "Population Control by Sterilization: The Cases of Puerto Rican and Mexican-Origin Women in the United States," *Latino(a) Research Review* 7, no. 3 (2009): 85–100.

43 Jessica Jaiswal, "Whose Responsibility Is It to Dismantle Medical Mistrust? Future Directions for Researchers and Health Care Providers," *Behavioral Medicine* 45, no. 2 (April 3, 2019): 188–96, https://doi.org/10.1080/08964289.2019.1630357.

44 Carl Kendall et al., "Understanding Pregnancy in a Population of Inner-City Women in New Orleans—Results of Qualitative Research," *Social Science & Medicine* 60, no. 2 (January 2005): 297–311, https://doi.org/10.1016/j.socscimed.2004.05.007.

45 Adam Tamburin, "Federal Court Order Officially Ends Tennessee 'Inmate Sterilization' Program," *The Tennessean*, May 20, 2019, www.tennessean.com.

46 Corey G. Johnson, "Female Inmates Sterilized in California Prisons without Approval," *Reveal*, July 7, 2013, https://revealnews.org; Anu Manchikanti Gomez, Liza Fuentes, and Amy Allina, "Women or LARC First? Reproductive Autonomy and the Promotion of Long-Acting Reversible Contraceptive Methods," *Perspectives on Sexual and Reproductive Health* 46, no. 3 (September 2014): 171–75, https://doi.org/10.1363/46e1614.

47 Caitlin Dickerson, Seth Freed Wessler, and Miriam Jordan, "ICE Detainees in Georgia Say They Had Unneeded Surgeries," *New York Times*, September 29, 2020, www.nytimes.com.

48 Roberts, *Killing the Black Body*.

49 Emily S. Mann and Patrick R. Grzanka, "Agency-Without-Choice: The Visual Rhetorics of Long-Acting Reversible Contraception Promotion," *Symbolic Interaction* 41, no. 3 (2018): 334–56, https://doi.org/10.1002/symb.349.

50 Leslie King and Madonna Harrington Meyer, "The Politics of Reproductive Benefits: US Insurance Coverage of Contraceptive and Infertility Treatments," *Gender & Society* 11, no. 1 (1997): 8–30.

51 For an in-depth historical analysis of the connection of racial science and trans medicine, see Emmett Harsin Drager, "Early Gender Clinics, Transsexual Etiology, and the Racialized Family," *GLQ: A Journal of Lesbian and Gay Studies* 29, no. 1 (January 1, 2023): 13–26, https://doi.org/10.1215/10642684-10144364.

52 J. Edgar Bauer, "Sexuality and Its Nuances: On Magnus Hirschfeld's Sexual Ethnology and China's Sapiential Heritage," *Anthropological Notebooks* 17, no. 1 (2011): 5–27, https://anthropological-notebooks.zrc-sazu.si/.

53 Sabine Lang, "Various Kinds of Two-Spirit People: Gender Variance and Homosexuality in Native American Communities," in *Two-Spirit People: Native American Gender Identity, Sexuality, and Spirituality*, ed. Sue-Ellen Jacobs,

Wesley Thomas, and Sabine Lang (Chicago: University of Illinois Press, 1997), 100–118.

54 Stryker, *Transgender History*.

55 Julian Gill-Peterson, *Histories of the Transgender Child* (Minneapolis: University of Minnesota Press, 2018).

56 Magnus Hirschfeld, "The Transvestites," in *The Transgender Studies Reader, ed. Susan Stryker and Stephen Wittle (New York: Routledge, 2006)*, 28–39.

57 Jordan D. Frey et al., "A Historical Review of Gender-Affirming Medicine: Focus on Genital Reconstruction Surgery," *Journal of Sexual Medicine* 14, no. 8 (2017): 991–1002.

58 Stryker, *Transgender History*, 40.

59 Stryker, 39.

60 Kami Horton, "Meet Oregonian Dr. Alan Hart, Who Underwent the First Documented Gender-Confirming Surgery in the US," Oregon Public Radio, June 30, 2022, www.opb.org.

61 J. Allen Gilbert, "Homo-Sexuality and Its Treatment," *Journal of Nervous and Mental Disease* 52, no. 4 (1920): 320.

62 Gilbert, 321.

63 Stryker, *Transgender History*.

64 West California Penal Code § 203 (n.d.).

65 *Barton v. State*, 282 S.W.2d 237 (n.d.).

66 John P. Holloway, "Transsexuals: Legal Considerations," *Archives of Sexual Behavior* 3, no. 1 (1974): 33–50.

67 Harry Benjamin, "The Transsexual Phenomenon," *Transactions of the New York Academy of Sciences* 29, no. 4, ser. 2 (1967): 428–30.

68 *Anonymous v. Weiner*, 270 N.Y.S.2d 319 (1966).

69 Lin Fraser, "Gender Dysphoria: Definition and Evolution through the Years," in *Management of Gender Dysphoria: A Multidisciplinary Approach*, ed. Carlo Trombetta, Giovanni Liguori, and Michele Bertolotto (Milan: Springer Milan, 2015), 19–31, https://doi.org/10.1007/978-88-470-5696-1_3.

70 Joanne J. Meyerowitz, *How Sex Changed* (Cambridge, MA: Harvard University Press, 2009).

71 Meyerowitz.

72 N. A. Bogoraz, "On Complete Plastic Reconstruction of a Penis Sufficient for Coitus," *Soviet Surgery* 8, no. 8 (1936): 303–9.

73 Matthew D. Freeman, Jared M. Gopman, and C. Andrew Salzberg, "The Evolution of Mastectomy Surgical Technique: From Mutilation to Medicine," *Gland Surgery* 7, no. 3 (June 2018): 308–15, https://doi.org/10.21037/gs.2017.09.07.

74 Milou Cecilia Madsen et al., "Testosterone in Men with Hypogonadism and Transgender Males: A Systematic Review Comparing Three Different Preparations," *Endocrine Connections* 11, no. 8 (June 27, 2022): e220112, https://doi.org/10.1530/EC-22-0112.

CHAPTER 2. WHY WOULD SOMEONE WANT A HYSTERECTOMY?

1 Brian Olshansky et al., "Postural Orthostatic Tachycardia Syndrome (POTS): A Critical Assessment," *Progress in Cardiovascular Diseases* 63, no. 3 (2020): 263–70, https://doi.org/10.1016/j.pcad.2020.03.010; Christine A. Varner, "Dysautonomia: Getting a Handle on POTS," *Nursing Made Incredibly Easy* 18, no. 4 (2020): 16–20.

2 Seth G. Derman, "Endometriosis," in *Encyclopedia of Endocrine Diseases*, ed. Luciano Martini (New York: Elsevier, 2004), 20–23, https://doi.org/10.1016/B0-12-475570-4/00433-9.

3 Clarke et al., "Biomedicalization."

4 Clarke et al., 214.

5 Elson, *Am I Still a Woman?*.

6 Hayley Braun et al., "Cancer in Transgender People: Evidence and Methodological Considerations," *Epidemiologic Reviews* 39, no. 1 (January 2017): 93–107, https://doi.org/10.1093/epirev/mxw003.

7 World Professional Association for Transgender Health, "Standards of Care."

8 Andréa Becker, "'Why Would We Take Men? This Is an OB/GYN': Gender, Hysterectomy, and the Patriarchal Dividend," *Sociology Compass* 17, no. 11 (November 2023): e13158, https://doi.org/10.1111/soc4.13158.

9 stef m. shuster, "Performing Informed Consent in Transgender Medicine," *Social Science & Medicine* 226 (2019): 190–97; Davis, Dewey, and Murphy, "Giving Sex."

10 Qiwei Yang et al., "Comprehensive Review of Uterine Fibroids: Developmental Origin, Pathogenesis, and Treatment," *Endocrine Reviews* 43, no. 4 (August 1, 2022): 678–719, https://doi.org/10.1210/endrev/bnab039; Derman, "Endometriosis."

CHAPTER 3. WHO CAN "CHOOSE" HYSTERECTOMY?

1 Waggoner, *Zero Trimester*.

2 Leeners et al., "Effect of Pregnancy on Endometriosis—Facts or Fiction?"

3 Alberico et al., "Potential Benefits of Pregnancy on Endometriosis Symptoms."

4 Elizabeth G. Raymond and David A. Grimes, "The Comparative Safety of Legal Induced Abortion and Childbirth in the United States," *Obstetrics & Gynecology* 119, no. 2, pt. 1 (February 2012): 215–19, https://doi.org/10.1097/

AOG.ob013e31823fe923; Evelyn J Patterson, Andréa Becker, and Darwin A. Baluran, "Gendered Racism on the Body: An Intersectional Approach to Maternal Mortality in the United States," *Population Research and Policy Review* 41, no. 3 (2022): 1261–94.

5 Maria Szubert et al., "Adenomyosis and Infertility—Review of Medical and Surgical Approaches," *International Journal of Environmental Research and Public Health* 18, no. 3 (February 2021): 1235, https://doi.org/10.3390/ijerph18031235; Damaris Freytag et al., "Uterine Fibroids and Infertility," *Diagnostics* 11, no. 8 (August 12, 2021): 1455, https://doi.org/10.3390/diagnostics11081455; Suneeta Senapati and Kurt Barnhart, "Managing Endometriosis-Associated Infertility," *Clinical Obstetrics and Gynecology* 54, no. 4 (December 2011): 720–26, https://doi.org/10.1097/GRF.ob013e3182353e06.

6 Michele G. Sullivan, "New Treatment Approved for Endometriosis Pain," *Family Practice News*, May 2005, 42a–42b, https://cdn.mdedge.com.

7 Becker, "'Why Would We Take Men? This Is an OB/GYN.'"

8 Nik M. Lampe, Shannon K. Carter, and J. E. Sumerau, "Continuity and Change in Gender Frames: The Case of Transgender Reproduction," *Gender & Society* 33, no. 6 (December 1, 2019): 865–87, https://doi.org/10.1177/0891243219857979.

9 Chris A. Barcelos, "'Bye-Bye Boobies': Normativity, Deservingness and Medicalisation in Transgender Medical Crowdfunding," *Culture, Health & Sexuality* 21, no. 12 (2019): 1–15.

10 Austin H. Johnson, "Transnormativity: A New Concept and Its Validation through Documentary Film about Transgender Men," *Sociological Inquiry* 86, no. 4 (2016): 465–91, https://doi.org/10.1111/soin.12127.

CHAPTER 4. HOW DO PEOPLE FEEL ABOUT HYSTERECTOMY?

1 Rene Almeling and Iris L. Willey, "Same Medicine, Different Reasons: Comparing Women's Bodily Experiences of Producing Eggs for Pregnancy or for Profit," *Social Science & Medicine* 188 (September 1, 2017): 21–29, https://doi.org/10.1016/j.socscimed.2017.06.027.

2 Lock and Kaufert, "Menopause, Local Biologies, and Cultures of Aging."

3 Lock and Kaufert.

4 Thakar, "Is the Uterus a Sexual Organ?"

5 Laura Mamo, *Queering Reproduction: Achieving Pregnancy in the Age of Technoscience* (Durham, NC: Duke University Press, 2007).

6 Gretchen Sisson, *Relinquished: The Politics of Adoption and the Privilege of American Motherhood* (New York: St. Martin's Press, 2024).

7 López, *Matters of Choice.*

CHAPTER 5. NAVIGATING ACCESS TO HYSTERECTOMY

1 Kathleen Broussard and Andréa Becker, "Self-Removal of Long-Acting Reversible Contraception: A Content Analysis of YouTube Videos," *Contraception* 104, no. 6 (December 1, 2021): 654–58, https://doi.org/10.1016/j.contraception.2021.08.002.

2 Heidi Moseson et al., "Self-Managed Abortion: A Systematic Scoping Review," *Best Practice & Research Clinical Obstetrics & Gynaecology* 63 (February 2020): 87–110, https://doi.org/10.1016/j.bpobgyn.2019.08.002.

3 Julia Neuberger, "Do We Need a New Word for Patients?," *BMJ: British Medical Journal* 318, no. 7200 (June 26, 1999): 1756–58.

4 Kelly Underman, *Feeling Medicine: How the Pelvic Exam Shapes Medical Training* (New York: New York University Press, 2020), 25.

5 Terri Kapsalis, *Public Privates: Performing Gynecology from Both Ends of the Speculum* (Durham, NC: Duke University Press, 1997), 6.

6 Underman, *Feeling Medicine*

7 Stefan Timmermans, "The Engaged Patient: The Relevance of Patient-Physician Communication for Twenty-First-Century Health," *Journal of Health and Social Behavior* 61, no. 3 (2020): 259–73.

8 Hege K. Andreassen and Marianne Trondsen, "The Empowered Patient and the Sociologist," *Social Theory & Health* 8, no. 3 (2010): 280–87.

9 Leo G. Reeder, "The Patient-Client as a Consumer: Some Observations on the Changing Professional-Client Relationship," *Journal of Health and Social Behavior* 13, no. 4 (1972): 406–12.

10 Shim, "Cultural Health Capital."

11 "LUPRON DEPOT® (Leuprolide Acetate for Depot Suspension)," LUPRON DEPOT, accessed August 31, 2023, www.luprongyn.com.

12 Verta Taylor and Lisa Leitz, "Emotions and Identity in Self-Help Movements," *Social Movements and the Transformation of American Health Care*, ed. Sandra Levisky (New York: Oxford University Press, 2010), 266–83.

13 Lauren Vogel, "Dr. YouTube Will See You Now," *Canadian Medical Association. Journal* 183, no. 6 (April 5, 2011): 647–48; Broussard and Becker, "Self-Removal of Long-Acting Reversible Contraception."

14 Jennifer A. Reich, "Teaching Women to Question and Control: Public Pedagogies of Birth and Vaccine Refusal," *BioSocieties* 15, no. 4 (2020): 580–600.

15 Bonham, "Race, Ethnicity, and Pain Treatment."

16 On fractures, see Knox H. Todd et al., "Ethnicity and Analgesic Practice," *Annals of Emergency Medicine* 35, no. 1 (January 1, 2000): 11–16, https://doi.

org/10.1016/S0196-0644(00)70099-0. On appendicitis, see Monika K. Goyal et al., "Racial Disparities in Pain Management of Children with Appendicitis in Emergency Departments," *JAMA Pediatrics* 169, no. 11 (November 1, 2015): 996–1002, https://doi.org/10.1001/jamapediatrics.2015.1915.

17 Kelly M. Hoffman et al., "Racial Bias in Pain Assessment and Treatment Recommendations, and False Beliefs about Biological Differences between Blacks and Whites," *Proceedings of the National Academy of Sciences* 113, no. 16 (April 19, 2016): 4296–301, https://doi.org/10.1073/pnas.1516047113.

18 Shim, "Cultural Health Capital."

CONCLUSION

1 Waggoner, *Zero Trimester*.

2 Anuradha Kumar, Leila Hessini, and Ellen M. H. Mitchell, "Conceptualising Abortion Stigma," *Culture, Health & Sexuality* 11, no. 6 (2009): 625–39.

3 Gross, *Vagina Obscura*.

4 Ballard, Lowton, and Wright, "What's the Delay?"; Dmowski et al., "Changing Trends in the Diagnosis of Endometriosis."

5 Raymond and Grimes, "Comparative Safety of Legal Induced Abortion and Childbirth in the United States."

6 Ushma D. Upadhyay et al., "Effectiveness and Safety of Telehealth Medication Abortion in the USA," *Nature Medicine* 30 (2024): 1–8.

7 Leah R. Koenig et al., "The Role of Telehealth in Promoting Equitable Abortion Access in the United States: Spatial Analysis," *JMIR Public Health and Surveillance* 9, no. 1 (November 7, 2023): e45671, https://doi.org/10.2196/45671.

8 Andréa Becker, "Elon Musk's Feud with Grimes Is a Warning," *Slate*, October 16, 2023, https://slate.com/technology/2023/10/elon-musk-grimes-babies-pronatalism-research.html.

APPENDIX

1 Allison J. Pugh, "What Good Are Interviews for Thinking about Culture? Demystifying Interpretive Analysis," *American Journal of Cultural Sociology* 1, no. 1 (2013): 42–68.

2 stef m. shuster, *Trans Medicine: The Emergence and Practice of Treating Gender* (New York: New York University Press, 2021).

3 Charlie Parker, Sam Scott, and Alistair Geddes, "Snowball Sampling," in *Sage Research Methods Foundations*, ed. Paul Atkinson, Sara Delamont, Alexandru Cernat, Joseph W. Sakshaug, and Richard A. Williams (London: Sage, 2019), https://doi.org/10.4135/9781526421036831710.

4   Stefan Timmermans and Iddo Tavory, "Theory Construction in Quali-
    tative Research: From Grounded Theory to Abductive Analysis," *So-
    ciological Theory* 30, no. 3 (September 1, 2012): 167–86, https://doi.
    org/10.1177/0735275112457914.

5   Kathy Charmaz, *Constructing Grounded Theory: A Practical Guide through
    Qualitative Analysis* (Thousand Oaks, CA: Sage, 2006).

INDEX

ABOUT THE AUTHOR

Andréa Becker is Assistant Professor in the Department of Sociology at Hunter College-CUNY. Her writing has appeared in the *New York Times*, *The Nation*, and *Slate*.